How Can I
Help?

Foreword by Paul F. Levy,
President and CEO of Beth Israel Deaconess Medical Center

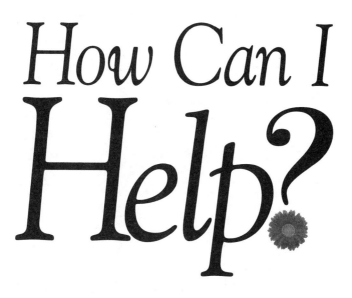

How Can I Help?

Everyday Ways to Help Your
Loved Ones Live with Cancer

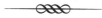

MONIQUE DOYLE SPENCER

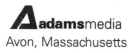

Avon, Massachusetts

Copyright © 2008, Monique Doyle Spencer
All rights reserved.
This book, or parts thereof, may not be reproduced in any
form without permission from the publisher; exceptions are
made for brief excerpts used in published reviews.

Published by
Adams Media, an F+W Publications Company
57 Littlefield Street, Avon, MA 02322. U.S.A.
www.adamsmedia.com

ISBN 10: 1-59869-681-5
ISBN 13: 978-1-59869-681-3

Printed in the United States of America.

J I H G F E D C B A

Library of Congress Cataloging-in-Publication Data
is available from the publisher.

This publication is designed to provide accurate and authoritative information
with regard to the subject matter covered. It is sold with the understanding that
the publisher is not engaged in rendering legal, accounting, or other professional
advice. If legal advice or other expert assistance is required, the services of a
competent professional person should be sought.

—From a *Declaration of Principles* jointly adopted by a Committee of the
American Bar Association and a Committee of Publishers and Associations

Many of the designations used by manufacturers and sellers to distinguish their
product are claimed as trademarks. Where those designations appear in this book
and Adams Media was aware of a trademark claim, the designations have been
printed with initial capital letters.

How Can I Help? is intended as a reference volume only, not as a medical manual.
In light of the complex, individual, and specific nature of health problems, this
book is not intended to replace professional medical advice. The ideas, procedures, and suggestions in this book are intended to supplement, not replace, the
advice of a trained medical professional. Consult your physician before adopting
the suggestions in this book, as well as about any condition that may require diagnosis or medical attention. The author and publisher disclaim any liability arising
directly or indirectly from the use of this book.

This book is available at quantity discounts for bulk purchases.
For information, please call 1-800-289-0963.

To
Mom and Dad
Sully and Doc

∽

And with grateful thanks to Eric Lupfer
of the William Morris Agency

Contents

� ❧

Contents

Acknowledgments

I AM GRATEFUL to so many people for their help in creating this book, especially my project team at Adams Media. But in learning the lessons of friendship, there's nobody quite like your siblings as teachers. They create the foundation of so many relationships in your life. We can hope that the adult relationships have no tattling, pushing, borrowing sweaters, hiding homework, or feeding your lunch to the dog. Still, it all starts at home.

I'm so glad that this book gives me the unique chance to thank my first best friends, my brothers and sisters:

Agnes Gootee
Denise Hughes
Mary "Mike" Williams
Thérèse (Terri) Grattan
Robert Doyle
Colette Doyle
Frank Doyle

Foreword

How MANY TIMES have you warmly and caringly said to a friend with cancer, "Call me if you need anything"? If you are like many other kind and considerate people, you are probably answering, "Lots of times." And having offered help in this manner, how many times have you actually been called? If you are like many other kind and considerate people, you are probably answering, "Gee, not very often." Maybe you figure that your friend did not need much help, or else he or she would surely have called. Maybe you have an inkling of doubt, though, and a twinge of guilt that you are not being as helpful as you think.

Now, let's turn the tables. Imagine you have been diagnosed with cancer. You are at some stage in your treatment process—surgery, radiation, or chemotherapy—and you are wondering if the treatment is going to work and how long you will have to live. You might also be feeling physically weak, or tired, or nauseated. You might not have much appetite. A kind and considerate friend pays a visit or calls on the phone and leaves you with the following message just before leaving or hanging up: "Call me if you need anything."

A show stopper. Later, if I am the patient, I am thinking about whether I will live to see my child's eighth-grade show. I remember that my friend said, "Call me if you need anything." Or, I am wondering if I will ever again enjoy the pungent smell of curry, and I think of my friend saying, "Call me if you need anything." I realize, when I drop my sock on the floor getting dressed, that I am in too much pain to bend over, and I recall that my friend said, "Call me if you need anything."

Somehow the words become a mocking shadow of their intended message. I *need* many things, but nothing you can offer me. I *need* many things, but you have to be here with me when I need them. I *need* many things, but I didn't know what I needed until you were long gone. A warm and caring expression leads me to despair.

Monique Doyle Spencer helps us understand that the kindest words in the world can impart unintended cruelty if we are not attuned to the mental and physical state of our friend with cancer. But she also knows that we are not cruel, that we are kind and caring and really want to be helpful to our friend in need. In the pages that follow she teaches us how to do this. In so doing, Monique often makes us laugh about cancer. She knows that laughter can help a cancer patient if it is employed at the right time in the treatment process. This book will help patients for that reason alone. But Monique's dry humor also succeeds in imparting wisdom to us friends-of-patients. It breaks down some of our own fear of this disease and lets us empathize with our friend. It also gives us common ground to laugh together with our friend and work on fighting the disease together.

Monique provides us with a cookbook of recipes that enable us to be helpful to cancer patients. She tells us how to say things that impart the right message, and she tells us how to do things that are truly useful and timely. She knows and trusts that we really do care, and she trains us how to deliver the goods and the good to our friends in need.

Paul F. Levy
President and Chief Executive Officer
Beth Israel Deaconess Medical Center
Boston, MA

Introduction

I HATE TO start you off in the ladies' room, but that's where this story begins. A woman is sobbing in the stall next to me. We're in the cancer wing, so she's probably not crying about the empty roll. I have to say something comforting.

"I know this is hard . . . ," I say.

She replies, "I'm going to smack that woman!"

I know what's coming. "She's my best friend. She has cancer. I want to help her. But I can't sit here all day while she sleeps through chemo! She should be up and walking! She would feel so much better if she would exercise! Every once in a while she wakes up and says she's uncomfortable, but she looks mighty comfortable to me in that recliner! I'm a terrible person." The sobbing begins again.

One good rule in life is to share nothing in ladies' rooms, like mascara, lip-gloss, or advice. But this was a very clear case. I knew what she needed.

"You took the wrong assignment," I tell her. "You're one of those people who can't sit still. You should be running errands, picking up kids, walking the dog. You're all wrong for the chemo buddy business. Fire yourself and give yourself a different job."

I hear a sniffle and a laugh.

Meanwhile, Over in Chemo . . .

Her friend, the patient, is napping fitfully. She's having a nightmare. Her gym teacher at Our Lady of Clinical Depression is yelling at her to run faster. She's supposed to run 2,500 meters but can't remember what a meter is, having been born before Americans went to Europe and came back eating funny cheese and speaking metric.

Her chemo buddy reminds her a lot of that gym teacher. She loves her friend but was relieved she went to the ladies' room. "If that woman tells me to get up and walk one more time I'll take this IV tube and wrap it around her neck." She jolts awake. Her friend is back. The two women look at each other and start to cry, or laugh, a little of both. "This is a disaster," they both say at once.

"Please let me go do errands for you," says the Sobber.

"I would love it if you could put food in my house for the kids," says the Patient, who knows she needs to be specific.

The Patient writes out a list, including some easy frozen entrees and treats.

The space-time continuum has been restored; all's right with the world. "Do you suppose Oprah and Gayle go through this?" asks the Cancer Patient.

The truly good friend would never get cancer, of course. It's a major inconvenience for everyone involved. In your lifetime, however, you're going to know at least one someone who has cancer. You want to help, but have no idea how. What should you say or not say? Should you ask about their chances of survival? Should you bring food? Should you offer a prayer group? Should you tell a cancer patient her wig is on sideways?

So, How Can You Help?

In speeches and interviews about my first book *The Courage Muscle: A Chicken's Guide to Living with Breast Cancer*, I hear one constant question: "How can I help my friend, sibling, parent, child, spouse, neighbor, coworker, boss, or employee while they cope with cancer?" If the audience includes cancer patients, there is a second standard question: "How do I handle it when people say or do awful things?"

That is the two-way street of cancer. It's designed by the same people who built the Los Angeles freeway system.

Cancer patients have a universal experience: Friends and family will carry them through thick and thicker—and family and friends will drive them crazy and make everything worse. Most cancer patients have loved ones who support them, but they also have the intrusive coworker, the friend who can't stand to hear the news and avoids contact, and the busybody who regales everyone with horror stories of other cancer patients, just as she once did about childbirth (which she never actually experienced, but still). Then there's the neighbor who can't keep any news to herself, who will tell so many people so much about you that it's all people can talk about when you run into them. At a time of greatest vulnerability, it's hard for cancer patients to cope with this extra burden. This book will offer simple ways to understand this problem and deal with it in ways to suit individual personalities.

On the other side of this two-way street, you're a friend who wants to help. First, what do you need to know about cancer? It's helpful to your friend if you know the basics about cancer and its treatment. The chances are high that the patient will survive, but it's a very bumpy road. The surgeries, the chemotherapy, the radiation, and the fear are hard to endure and hard to watch.

Even though we all know someone with cancer, living or dead, we are often struck with silence when we hear the news. We don't know what to say, we don't know how to help, and sometimes we're nervous about seeing the person at all. Countless caring people fear that they will say or do the wrong thing.

I was first diagnosed with stage III breast cancer in 2001, so I've seen a lot of people in treatment and a lot of people who love them. Patients and friends are equally new at this, and both start off with few skills. Both need help. We'll start off with a basic understanding of cancer, just enough information so that you can understand what is happening to your friend.

Chapter One

Cancer 101

❧

YOUR FRIEND HAS just been diagnosed with cancer. Emotionally, this is the very worst part. She really will feel better and happy again, but right now she feels like the gates of hell are yawning open at her front door. Stick by her, let her wallow for a little while; she's going to come out of this. There's just no rushing it. She's got to get her mind around this and figure out how she's going to handle it. For many people, that takes a month and often longer.

In the meantime, it's going to be a roller coaster. There will be days of quiet strength, to be sure, but plenty of other days of fear. The worst fear is among diagnosed parents of young children. At this stage, many people assume they're going to die, and they picture every milestone in the children's lives that they're going to miss. The thought of grandchildren will start a torrent. Most cancer patients will tell you that this is the one part of cancer that brought him or her to their knees. The only way through this stage is straight through it, as with many challenges in life. There is no sentence you can say that is going to make life all better for your friend while she finds her way through the diagnosis stage. Be there for her and listen. Let her come to realize that *she's* the one whose life may be at risk—not the kids. *Sounds* crazy, but it feels so much better. The truth is that most people, by far, survive cancer. It just doesn't feel that way to your friend right now.

Stages of Cancer

After the diagnosis, there will be a bunch of tests to figure out how serious this is and what kind of treatment is going to be needed. These are mostly scans and blood tests. Some people really like company for these appointments. Some of the tests are quick, some take half a day. For bone scans, for example, patients go in first for some radioactive dye that has to work its way through their system. There will be several hours between the injection and the scan. Your friend might like company to go for a walk or coffee. (This is different from the bone density scan you might have had to screen for osteoporosis, which is quick.)

The doctor is trying to find what stage of cancer your friend has. Most cancers go from stage I up to stage IV. In breast cancer, there is also a stage 0, which is very small and early. It's helpful to know the stage, so suggest to your friend that she ask her doctor to explain it. The earlier the stage, the higher the chances for survival. It doesn't mean that later stages are the end, just that cancer is best treated when it is as new and as small as possible.

The staging system changes for each type of cancer, but usually tells us how much the cancer has grown and how far cancer cells have traveled from the original site. Some systems use letters instead of Roman numerals, other systems need completely different terms, such as for leukemia or lymphoma, which don't have a starting point like a solid tumor does. Here's a look at the staging that may be used for a solid tumor cancer such as breast cancer. *Remember to be sure that your friend has accurate information from the doctor about staging—some cancers have completely different methods!*

- Stage 0 is a small and very early cluster of cells that have the features of cancer cells, but they have not invaded anything yet. It is also called "in situ."
- Stage I means that the tumor is small. No lymph nodes are affected.

- Stage II means that the tumor is bigger or it has spread to lymph nodes.
- Stage III is when the tumor is bigger and cancer cells are found in the lymph nodes.
- Stage IV means that cancer cells have spread to other parts of the body.

I missed school the very sunny day in 1977 that we learned about lymph nodes. They're like little turkey basters and we have many of them. They take lymph, which is liquid that carries everything around the body, such as infection-fighting cells, and they squirt it from one part to another, in places like the groin and underarms. They can also send cancer cells along.

It's important to know if there are cancer cells in the lymph nodes because that's often the first place they go after starting a tumor. When cancer cells spread to other parts of your body, they're just like people who tear down small houses and build big ones. They multiply rapidly compared to the cells around them, and they take over that part of the body. That's what cancer is.

When someone has cancer that has spread to the lymph nodes, a surgeon will take out as many lymph nodes as necessary from the area. Many people have a "sentinel node" biopsy first. They put a little dye in and see where it goes. Usually, the lymph fluid goes to one node first, like a teacher who calls on the same kid all the time. They will look at this node and if it's cancer free, they can often assume that no other nodes are involved. If it's positive, though, they'll keep looking and removing.

Your friend's pathology report after surgery will have this information, at least: how big the tumor is, how aggressive the cancer is, and how many lymph nodes are involved. In some cancers, such as breast and prostate cancer, they will also look for hormone receptors; this means that the cancer feeds on hormones, and this information will help with treatment planning. The surgeon will likely talk about the "margins" around the tumor. They want to make sure that they took a nice clean border around the tumor that had no cancer cells in it.

If your friend wants to see the report, he can ask for it. Be prepared that there will be at least a dozen scary-sounding words that mean nothing! But it can be useful to have this report if your friend is seeking a second opinion. Now he knows the stage.

Your Stage 0 or I Friend

This is a nice early stage with high survival rates. The doctor will say things like "If you could pick a cancer, this is the one to have," or "This is a good cancer."

It's true, nearly everybody survives early cancer. You'd think that would make it emotionally easy, but it doesn't. Your friend will have fear, and she'll likely be numb with shock. It may be early, but the doctor is still calling it "cancer." Early-stage treatment plans will depend on how aggressive the cancer cells are, the size, the type of cancer, and the age of the patient. And maybe the doctor's attorney. Medical malpractice suits have encouraged even very good doctors to give more aggressive treatments. The problem is that some early-stage patients will have recurrences later, but doctors don't know which ones. This is why making treatment decisions in early stages can drive your friend crazy.

For example, the early-stage patient usually does not have to have chemotherapy. Chemo may be no picnic, but it does make you feel that everything in the world is being done to stop the cancer. In fact, if no chemo is involved, patients in stages 0 and I may feel that they get a boo-boo kiss and a Band-Aid. They'll have the tumor or cancer cells removed, and radiation may be recommended, which can be challenging but not visibly so.

The problem? The patient is going to wonder if she should have aggressive treatment anyway, with the hope that she might prevent a future recurrence. She's going to agonize over it. Her family is going to become experts on it. And at the end of the day, she may as well toss a coin, because right now there is no way to tell who's going to have recurrences and who's not.

Support groups are filled with early-stage patients. I think it's because they're pretty much dismissed as "lucky." You can help an early-stage friend greatly by understanding that her fear is real. I think it would help early-stage patients if we had different words for early cancer and advanced cancer. To me, stage IV is what I think of as Cancer. Right now, whether a person has stage 0 or stage IV, the pathology report still says "carcinoma," which means cancer. It's hard to get that out of your head.

How Can You Best Help This Early-Stage Friend?

Offer a reasonable ear. A reasonable ear means that you listen without changing the subject or jumping in with your views.

Your next steps are going to vary greatly from friend to friend. Is she a person who has to understand everything in life? Did she read every pregnancy book ever written? That's what she's going to do now. She probably reads instruction manuals, too. You either love this about her or it drives you nuts, and that's not going to change. Everyone gets to choose a personal path through this.

You have to make your own way through this, too. If you're unable to stand hearing every detail of her research, choose another way to be a good friend. Do a favorite activity of hers; see the kind of movie she likes; go for the long walk she craves. If you're close friends, be direct about it. Don't just avoid her or the subject. Tell her that you're overwhelmed by information and you want to find a different way to help.

Your Stage II–III Friend

In the middle stages, II and III, the tumor has grown larger and/or the cancer cells have invaded the nearby lymph nodes. Stages II and III have a higher risk and usually require more aggressive treatment. The basic cancer treatment tools are surgery, chemotherapy, radiation, and antihormone therapy. Patients in stage II and III will likely have a combination of at least a few of those.

In stages II and III you begin to see what you think of as "cancer." Surgery may be more extensive—around the tumor and in the lymph nodes. The recovery may be more difficult and painful.

There's also a chance of developing lymphedema when lymph nodes and channels are removed, damaged, or radiated. Lymphedema can be a minor problem or a major one. It's a subject all by itself (see Appendix B: Helpful Resources). Just know that if your friend is having swelling in a limb where lymph nodes are missing, he should call the doctor. Help him by insisting.

In these middle stages, chemotherapy is likely. By the way, I am grouping stages II and III together because the treatment path is the same, even though there are differences in the size or extent of the cancer. It's a bit like bronchitis and pneumonia, where the illness is different but the medicine is often the same.

Chemotherapy is usually the major challenge of cancer treatment, but it varies so widely and wildly from person to person that nobody, including your friend's doctor, can predict exactly what's going to happen. The only accurate prediction is that your friend can count on some sick days, some fatigue, some days of just feeling tired, but the horror stories of chemotherapy twenty years ago no longer apply to most patients. Doctors offer many new treatments that minimize side effects.

How Can You Best Help This Middle-Stage Friend?

In stages II and III you begin to see what you think of as typical "cancer." The diagnosis stage will be the same as in all stages: You want to listen and give company and support.

Normally, the first step of diagnosis does not include staging. When the staging news comes in, there will usually be another bump of shock. For the pessimist, who was expecting to be staged at stage IV, stage II will be great news. To the optimistic ones who thought the original diagnosis must be a mistake, stage II is devastating. But in general, middle- and advanced-stage patients will feel the worst second shocks—and you'll want to be there for them.

Since recovery for these middle-stage patients may be more difficult and more painful, you'll want to start reaching into the toolboxes you'll find in Chapters 7 and 8.

Your Stage IV Friend

In stage IV, called metastatic cancer, the cells have spread to distant sites such as the lungs, bones, brain, or liver. This is the most challenging cancer. With metastatic cancer, the challenges are going to be lifelong, no matter how long that will be. For some, cancer is beaten. For some, death follows diagnosis within months. For many, life becomes a series of recurrences, surgeries, chemotherapy, and clinical trials. Cancer becomes a new part-time or even full-time job.

The challenges for friends and family can be immense. Generally, the group of supporters will grow smaller as the condition becomes a chronic illness. Try your very best to stick with your friend.

Some cancers, such as breast cancer, have such extensive early-detection tools that it's uncommon for a woman to hear "stage IV" at her very first diagnosis. Other cancers, such as pancreatic or ovarian, are silent. For this patient, the first diagnosis may be shocking. Your friend may be handed a life-threatening diagnosis; she has the real thing and is in for a seemingly overwhelming struggle.

The period of diagnosis is going to be intense for people with stage IV cancer. Read through what the earlier-stage cancer patients experience, triple the intensity, and you'll get the idea of what your friend is facing.

If you look up statistics for stage IV, you'll be frightened. Remem-

> **" I loved it when my friend . . . "**
>
> ". . . Took care of my kids."
>
> ". . . Waited for my kids at our rural school bus stop when I couldn't."
>
> ". . . Prayed for me."
>
> ". . . Prayed with me."
>
> ". . . Put my name on prayer lists."

ber a few things about these numbers. First, they're about people who were diagnosed five years ago. They're not about present-day treatment and your friend. *Every prognosis number you see, for every stage of every cancer, is based on old information, even on brand-new Web sites.* They take a group of patients and see how many are still alive five years later. Some of those patients were not as healthy as your friend, or maybe didn't finish treatment. There are new treatments, too. Those numbers include everyone who was diagnosed, and your friend might have better doctors, better resistance, better support. We should really have a stage V. As challenging as a stage IV diagnosis is, there are degrees of disease. Your friend may be living a full and long life, and it's important to understand that. For a wonderful discussion on cancer statistics, read the Stephen Jay Gould article recommended in the Helpful Resources appendix. He lived twenty years longer than he was supposed to!

For many stage IV patients today, cancer really is a chronic illness, not a death sentence. It's tough, exhausting, and scary, like diabetes and other chronic illnesses, but often with much more difficult treatments. Every stage IV patient struggles with the balance between spending time living versus spending time trying not to die. Treatments can take a lot of enjoyment out of life, and patients will have to decide how much they're willing to do. Many people decide to fight the medical fight until their last day. Many others decide to start traveling or taking cruises or getting a few things done, and they don't want to devote time to treatment.

Your friend is going to start hearing about clinical trials, which are tests of new treatments. Every cancer is different; he may find many clinical trials, in which he can try experimental drug treatments, or few. Check Appendix B at the end of the book for help. If your friend is treated at a medical center, chances are they're the ones running the trials. But check out what's happening at other hospitals, too. Sometimes even the best hospital doesn't happen to have the latest experiment running for your friend's kind of cancer. Clinical trials can be controversial, but the majority are good things. Just go in with questions and get opinions from your doctor and other people you respect.

Nobody can predict the outcome of your friend's choice to continue treatment, to find a clinical trial, or to stop treatment. Your friend might have difficult days surrounded by good days, or have nothing but bad days; she might gain many years of a normal life, or none. This is when you realize that the agonizing decisions of early cancer seem pretty minor in comparison.

How Can You Best Help Your Stage IV Friend?

Follow every step you did when your friend was first diagnosed. Listen like a dog. Think about her needs. Help her to live her life the way she dreamt it would be.

The unknowns for your friend are troubling during this time. She's asking herself: If I fight this, can I survive and live a few more years really well? Would I die soon if I don't? If I fight this, will the treatment weaken me? If it doesn't work, will I have wasted my time and regret it?

You love your friend, so she's going to ask your opinion. She's going to ask what you would do. Ask for time. Tell her you want to think about it and you'll get back to her, but in the meantime could she please tell you more about what she's thinking? Is she leaning one way or the other?

If anyone makes their life plans based on certain death, not chronic illness, they're going to run out of steam. Me, I would run out of money. Given a stage IV diagnosis, I would spend every penny I have, develop a drinking problem, start smoking, and engage in any unsafe activity I could think of. Then, to my horror, I'd keep waking up alive. Broke and alive.

Many people have thought the same. Having said that, everybody needs a real plan for the end of life. Our beloved Congressman Joe Moakley of South Boston, Massachusetts, who died of cancer, said that he didn't know how anybody dies "without three month's notice." You might be able to help your friend get those things done that we all put off, like a will. Do yours together maybe. It will make her feel that this is a normal responsibility.

❧

So that's the basic information you need to know about cancer. If this is your first experience up close, it probably still looks very blurry. The next chapter will give you a road map of what typically happens and when.

CARE ALERT

With this chapter and some Internet research, you may feel like an expert on cancer. Be cautious about that. If your friend has got a good medical team, don't flood her with information unless she asks you for it.

Chapter Two

Cancer Timeline:
What to Expect and How to Help

☙

YOU'RE ABOUT TO begin a journey with your friend; you have no idea where you're going or when it will end. There are many predictable milestones, though. So what will this process be like?

Diagnosis

In the first month of cancer, the patient may as well take his brain out and keep it in the freezer. He gets this news, he thinks he's going to die, he's grieving like a banshee, his life passes before his eyes really slowly, and it's mostly the bad bits. This is, by far, the hardest time for him and his mental state.

Patients need a few kinds of help during this time. They have to get their minds around cancer and what it's going to mean for them. They have to have a bunch of tests to find out if the cancer is spreading. They have to start planning their lives around treatment or surgery. It's a busy time, and to many cancer patients it's a blur.

How can you help? Take stock of yourself first—just like on a plane when you're supposed to put the oxygen mask on yourself first before assisting your children. Review what your strengths are and what you're not so good at. Can you be a calm helper, or are you still crying your head off every time you think about him? Does he need an organizer? (Which you're either good at or not!) Does he need somebody to take charge of rides? (And you either have a reliable and comfortable car or you don't!) Are you someone who's good at understanding medical stuff so he can get the basics of what's happening?

During this stage, it's hard for the cancer patient to believe that life will ever be good again. It's exactly, precisely like feeling seasick. He just knows he will never feel normal again. You can tell the patient over and over that he really will get through this, that life really will be great again—but his mind needs time. You can't rush it. Just encourage him to believe it.

My best friend, Laura, took the news matter-of-factly. I waited a while before I told her, because she was involved in planning a huge project and I didn't want to dampen it. When I did, she was calm, concerned, and practical. A year later, Laura admitted to me that she cried when she got off the phone.

How you feel about tears is so individual, but I was thankful she waited until we were off the phone. I wasn't crying about cancer, and I didn't have a lot of patience for people doing it around me. I think this tears thing depends on where your ancestors came from. You'll understand what I mean if you ever heard these words from your parents: "You're crying? I'll give you something to cry about!"

If tears help you, or if crying is your normal response, go ahead of course. Just don't be hurt if your friend tells you to go cry in the bathroom. This sounds harsh, I know. It's just that many patients don't want to view their situations as tragedies. Tears say "grief" to many people. Tears may also make your friend feel that he has to comfort *you*, which is not why you're there to help.

Spreading the News

Everybody chooses their own way to tell friends about cancer. I just got a group e-mail from a friend who said: "I have cancer. Please don't call me. I will e-mail you with any news." Few people are this blunt, but many people feel that way. They're overwhelmed and don't want to keep telling the story over and over.

What can you do? Send a card. Wait for an opening, if there is one. Eventually, if his situation is serious, he'll need help; so keep in touch. You may feel insulted that he doesn't want to see you yet. Remember: This is a sign of exhaustion in him, not exclusion. Also, try to be understanding if you're not the first person who finds out that your friend has cancer. It means nothing.

There's no rhyme or reason to this stage. Some people call anyone they know who has had cancer first, so a neighbor hears before a friend. Some people tell total strangers for a few days, which is odd, but common. You don't care about the stranger so you tell them everything. Some people really dread calling the people they love the most. They tell the people at work before they tell the best friend or Mom and Dad. I've even heard someone on a plane confessing all medical details to the stranger next to them. Someone I know, who is not me, actually spoke at length about it, in English, to a manicurist who speaks only Vietnamese.

For me, calling my father was the hardest call of all. I dreaded it. No other call was so difficult. I felt that he deserved a free ride after my mother's death from cancer. He shouldn't have to worry about a child. For other people, calling Mom or Dad is the first step and the easiest.

We're all different, so as a friend, respect the manner in which your friend informs everyone—it's one of the few things he may feel like he actually has control over at the time.

Decisions about Treatment

Some patients have few decisions to make about treatment; some have many. This can be very complex, depending on the type of cancer. Breast cancer has many choices, especially about reconstruction. Some women agonize over every decision, some breeze through. Prostate cancer has many treatment options, from surgery to radiation to anti-hormone shots to "wait and see." As far as I can tell, prostate cancer has the most confusing and conflicting options of all cancers. It requires plenty of research and several opinions before the patient wants to make a decision.

Prostate cancer patients discover that many doctors have a personal idea on the subject, so that's what they offer. One of my friends was told to drop everything and come in for surgery. The next doctor said no surgery, just radiation. The next said do nothing. The next said antihormone treatment. These were all top-level doctors in major Boston teaching hospitals. They were all correct—these are reasonable approaches to prostate cancer. But these doctors did not tell my friend "here are four reasonable options"; they each only recommended one. So be sure your friend always asks what the alternatives are.

Oddly, early stage cancers are often the most confusing to make decisions about. If your friend is a stage III patient, he's very likely having chemotherapy. If he's stage I with no lymph node involvement, it's not so certain. And guess what? It may end up being his own decision.

I have listened to many friends go through this decision. My advice to them is to toss a coin. The patient can't figure out the right answer, because nobody can, including the doctor. So if it were me, I would just guess. Or hold a lottery.

Your friend will seek advice from people who have had treatment, particularly when it comes to chemo. This is a bit like asking a mother if you should have children. If you ask a woman in labor, she will not smile quietly and say yes. If you ask her the next morning, she will. She might be wrong both times.

So, people who have had chemo might advise for it or against it. Encourage your friend to focus on his own circumstances. His cancer may be early but aggressive, which changes the channel. Nobody can make this decision for him. Don't try.

Families and loved ones can be very pushy about treatment. They want the patient around for as long as possible. They think aggressive treatment is the answer, whether it's needed or not. Personally, I don't agree. I know a man who was diagnosed with prostate cancer at the age of seventy-five. His doctor advised him to do nothing. "You'll die with it, not of it," is the standard wisdom at that age.

The man's wife, however, was having none of that. She demanded that he be treated, *now*. The man thought she knew better than he did because she had medical training. So my friend spent an uncomfortable time in radiation, which he had a bad reaction to, and took a year to recover.

> **" I loved it when my friend . . . "**
>
> ". . . Listened to me."
>
> ". . . Listened to my spouse."
>
> ". . . Took my spouse out for a break."
>
> ". . . Listened to my parents."
>
> ". . . Drove my elderly parents so that they could visit me."

Researching Treatment Options

If your friend is the research type, there is an interesting tool offered by the American Cancer Society online. He can go to *www.cancer.org/profiletools* and click "Making Treatment Decisions."

Click on the type of cancer, then fill in the online questionnaire. They will ask about his age, the size of the tumor, if there is lymph node involvement, all of the basics. The tool generates a report of treatment options with detailed information on each one, including side effects.

If your friend really wants to go crazy, you can then click on "Treatment Outcomes." This section will give you studies on the statistics about different treatment combinations, meaning what impact the combination appears to have on survival.

This is no way to make a decision, needless to say. But it's a nifty tool and may give your friend some confidence in the doctor's plan. It's also a good place to read about the different types of treatment and review the information the doctor gave your friend (which your friend is likely to have already forgotten). It will also provide some questions to ask the doctor. The program is called the Nex-Profiler Treatment Option Tools for Cancer and *it's free*. If your friend thinks there's a problem with his treatment plan, offer to attend a meeting with the doctor with him. Encourage your friend to get a second opinion. Once he's decided, however, shut up.

Treatment

After reviewing treatment options comes the treatment. This could be surgery, reconstruction, chemotherapy, radiation, or antihormone treatment. In the next chapter we'll go into these treatments in detail, but it's good to start with a general understanding of what's ahead.

I view cancer treatment as a marathon in which somebody throws in a few hundred-yard dashes along the way. Throughout treatment, your body is trying to cope with major challenges that feel pretty constant and chronic, such as fatigue. That's the marathon part of it. But there are also spikes that are harder and they are a little different for everyone. Some people have a few bad days after each chemo treatment, some don't; some people have pain, some don't; some people breeze through a treatment, some don't. Just be prepared for change, and for the unexpected, because you can be sure there will be surprises along the way.

Posttreatment Blues

Posttreatment depression is as common as postnatal blues, but without all the baby gifts. It takes many forms, with obstacles to be overcome in order to return to a new but normal life.

The first obstacle is fear, and it's the most common. Some people can't stop thinking about cancer. They are gripped by fear. You can see it in their faces. While in treatment, they felt safe. Doctors and nurses surrounded them and it gave them the feeling that nothing could go wrong. Now they are feeling very alone. Every pain, every lump, causes panic. They imagine cancer cells floating around the bloodstream looking for the liver. I imagine it must be similar for someone who has heart disease and worries when they exercise.

Some people, honestly, miss the casseroles. They got used to being taken care of. Their coping muscles have atrophied and they don't want to go back to real life. Others miss the warm outpouring of affection. Cancer can be a time of great strain in a family, but it can also be a time of reconciliation and affection. You can be enveloped in unconditional love for the first time since you were a baby. You don't want to give it up for the conditional kind you usually get.

Some people have a hard time getting used to their new bodies. No matter how great a reconstructed body part is, it's still a substitute. Some people go on a years-long search for the perfect plastic surgeon to tinker with shapes, scars, or creases.

Some people struggle with the aftereffects of treatment. Chemo may have thrown them into early menopause, male or female. Antihormone drugs may do the same. Radiation may cause scarring, or lumps, or thickening. Some types of chemo can cause nerve damage in hands and feet that may or may not get better.

Some people, even if they don't have any physical side effects from treatment, just can't shake the cancer life. It used to be that when a person was finished with treatment, they were expected to shut up and feel better. Then the pendulum swung in the opposite direction. Now everyone is supposed to continue being sensitive to the patient, listening to them talk about and dwell on *cancer*. There is a melodrama to the whole experience that I think is unhealthy for everyone, patient and friend.

As the friend, I'm not advising you to be mean, of course. But all of the helpers need a break, and the patient needs to return to normal life. Delaying that return does not help. In my view, delaying that return causes depression. Inactivity does the same thing.

So what can you do? Tell the patient gently: "We all need and want you to be feeling better again. We want life to feel normal. That's hard for you, I know, but we'll get you there."

Don't expect your friend to jump back to normal on the last day of treatment, because his body won't and his mind won't either. It takes time. But if the emotional trend isn't generally upward, your friend is standing still in the world of cancer. He worries constantly, he feels for lumps more often than he showers, he's constantly reviewing his health for symptoms.

You can help your friend by making sure he has a long-term plan from his doctor. He should know how often he will be seen and what follow-up tests may be typically needed. He should know when he is supposed to call about a symptom. This planning makes it a little easier to "plan" when to worry! Your friend can work on confining worry to actual symptoms or checkups. That will still be worrying, but at least it's not consuming him. It is also helpful for you to know:

- What aftereffects of treatment are normal
- When your friend is supposed to call the doctor
- What his checkup schedule is
- What emotions he may be having that are normal and will go away

It is not helpful to keep him dependent on family and friends when he is physically healthy. You wouldn't do that for a friend with diabetes; don't do it for a cancer patient.

It cannot be overstated—encourage your friend to find the day when he can quit reading about cancer and start a new chapter of living. The solution, for many people, is to make a conscious choice every morning to appreciate every new day. For others, prayer helps. Faith helps. Work helps. Responsibilities help. For some, a support group or therapy will help.

Recurrence

It's possible that at some point after treatment, the cancer will return. If your friend is "lucky," it is a new local cancer and has not spread anywhere. This is technically called a new primary cancer and not a recurrence. In this case, the treatment plan is largely a repetition of what's come before. That will be challenging enough.

But recurrence can mean metastasis, which means, "spread." Some people say they have metastatic cancer when they have lymph node involvement, but usually metastasis means that the cancer cells have taken up residence someplace important—the bones, the lungs, the brain, the organs.

Life has just changed in a big way. Your friend will have many more tests, more treatments, more surgeries, more experiments. He will be flooded with advice from everyone who ever read a tabloid insisting that eating bark and giving up chocolate will save his life.

So what happens next? Treatment may be more of the same or it may be very different. When your friend is diagnosed with recurring cancer, you can encourage him to head for a medical center if he is not yet being treated at one. The community hospital, while wonderful, is usually not the place to go for advanced cancer treatment. They aren't staffed for that and they'll probably tell you that

themselves. Good doctors have no problem making referrals to experts when that is needed.

With metastatic recurrence, your friend needs to ask
everyone in the world where the best treatment is. His
doctor may know. His doctor can help to get appointments,
too. Don't accept any long waiting times for scheduling
appointments. The secret of doctor's appointments is this:
Doctors usually cannot bring themselves to turn anyone
away. They are healers and if people lined up for twenty-
four hours a day, they'd be there to take care of them. Since
that's impossible, they hire a front desk staff. The people in
charge of appointments will only tell you when the next
available one is, which will be in two months. Their job is
to protect the doctor from overscheduling. Your friend's job
is to find a way around that. His doctor can call or e-mail
and get past the front desk—if it's absolutely necessary.

Metastasis is going to test your friend, you, and your friendship in a whole new way. He may be unable to talk about anything else, which you may get tired of. You may be unable to
ask about anything else, which he may get tired of.

Follow the same steps you did for his earlier cancer. Take
stock of yourself and your resources. Listen. Provide what
you can, and do whatever you and he agree is most important. Know that this could be a very long haul and that you
need to pace yourself.

As you probably already know, treatment of metastatic cancer has come a long way. It used to be a death sentence, and for many people it still is. For an increasing number, however, it has become what your doctor will call a "chronic" illness, not a terminal one.

This means that your friend is likely to have a few battles ahead, because his cancer is not curable. There may be more recurrences, surgeries, treatments, all of which can give him a high-quality and long life, but are still challenging.

> **"I loved it when my friend . . . "**
>
> ". . . Expected me to be normal most of the time."
>
> ". . . Called my parents when I was out of it just to give upbeat reports."
>
> ". . . Brought a pile of fabulous fabrics over and taught me to wrap my bald and cold head with them, African style."
>
> ". . . Took me to treatments."
>
> ". . . Took care of me during treatments—getting drinks, food, magazines."

You will be friends for a long time, or you wouldn't be reading this book, and his challenges may develop over many years. Many people, when cancer first metastasizes, actually have few symptoms. Treatment will begin right away anyway, but your friend may actually be feeling fine. It's a strange sensation and it's going to take him some time to figure this out, to get his mind around it.

He is facing a major mental challenge: How do you live your life with metastatic cancer? Let's say he is feeling well, and strong, and he has responsibilities. At the same time there is a great big bump in the road and it's hard not to spend all of his time thinking about that.

People who have metastatic cancer often say that after the initial period of shock and grief, they began to develop this goal: to have cancer be part of your life without *being* your life. They train themselves to focus on cancer when they have to—during treatment or testing—and to focus on "real life" otherwise. Getting to this point can take a month or many months, and you can help your friend by reminding him that diagnosis is the worst stage and that he will eventually figure this out.

Spend time together doing ordinary things. Talk about the same things you've always talked about. In other words, keep practicing your normal friendship! The more you help him maintain as normal a routine as possible, the more control he will have of his thoughts. "Practicing" helps people to avoid obsessing.

Still, you'll have to decide how you will handle your own emotional challenges. What if he is your best friend and you are grieving terribly that he is sick again? What if he is the friend you would normally go to for help with grief?

It can be a big adjustment, but you will probably have to search for someone else to help comfort you. I'm not telling you never to express your grief to your friend, just that he will likely not have the emotional resources to be of much help. He's going to have to reserve that energy for his children and siblings.

You will find that every patient differs in how they want to view the future. Some people want to anticipate the worst possible outcome and plan ahead, still hoping that they will beat this. Others like to believe that nothing bad is going to happen and they will appear to have forgotten they have a recurrence! Most fall somewhere in between, and most change their outlook over time. Many even change over the course of a single day. This is another time when your listening skills will come in very handy.

If Nothing Helps

There are cases of cancer that can't be treated and can't be stopped. Nobody can help. You may feel the same way about your grief when you learn that your friend is unlikely to survive. There is no cure for you, either. I'll share some thoughts with you, because I do know one thing:

Eventually, as with all crises, life is going to go on, and you will eventually be able to cope with your grief.

Let's start with the idea of dying. When you have stood and looked over that cliff, or stood there with a dear friend, you might come to the belief that many of us do: that there is no such thing as "dying," except in the last few days or so of illness. You are either alive or dead, and there's nothing in between. At the end of life, most of us don't want to feel that we are spending our time dying—we want to spend it living.

Whatever you and your friend believe about the afterlife, this journey is an important part of his life. It's a journey everybody has to make. He is doing it sooner than he should have to, but it is still important that he craft his journey the way he wants it to be.

Why is that important to know? Because you'll have plenty of time to grieve later. Right now, he is living and you can too.

I also know that when sick people reach the moment of death, they rarely look afraid. We fear death, most of us, but people who are a minute away from it are generally at a much different place.

How do you help if it comes to the end of life? Focus on comfort. Foot rubs, gentle massages, cool cloths, warm comforters, fresh air, aromatherapy, music, prayer, whatever seems to make the patient comfortable. Bring some comfortable chairs into his room for visitors. (Or if he doesn't want long visits, remove the chairs!) The point is that there is always something you can do to make your friend's *life* a little bit better. Many people love the sound of conversation and laughter, even if they don't appear to hear it or understand it.

Often, at the end of life, the family will arrive from around the country to be with your friend, praying, holding a kind of vigil. This can be hard for you if you don't feel welcome here. We've all seen it happen—the loyal friend who has been there through it all is pushed aside at the deathbed by the bossy daughter-in-law.

What can you do, especially when you are pushed aside? First, think food! Bring some basic supplies to your friend's room. Water bottles, napkins, sandwiches, all low-odor, low-fuss things. By making things comfortable for a grieving family, you are helping your friend in a deeply loving way.

You might also schedule your visits when the family goes off to sleep. In the last days of a dear friend's life, pulling up a rocking chair and even dozing off as you say a few prayers can be of great comfort to both of you.

Hospice and Palliative Care

Hospice and palliative care are nearly the same thing. Palliative care is provided to patients who are seriously ill but may or may not be terminally ill. It may or may not be covered by insurance. Hospice care refers to care provided in the last six months of life after a diagnosis of terminal disease and is often covered.

The concept of both programs is the same: Seriously or terminally ill patients should receive care and comfort even when there is no cure. They should be relieved of pain. They should be spared invasive, unnecessary procedures or tests. Their families should be comforted, during the last months of life and through grieving.

How is it different from regular nursing? It simplifies care. Hospice workers can provide medicine without the layers of approval needed in the traditional hospital setting. If a doctor in the hospital prescribes pain relief every four hours, the nurses cannot change that without the doctor's approval. In the middle of the night on a summer weekend, your friend may wait far too long. The hospice worker can typically give pain relief as needed.

Most people think this kind of care is great under these trying circumstances. Hospice workers come to the home or wherever the patient is living. They can help to give the patient comfort and can help the family to navigate the end of life. So it's not just that they tend to be nice people who are willing to spend their time in situations like this. They can make a big difference in your friend's comfort.

I visited a man whose wife would not sign him up for hospice. She seemed to think that to do so would be giving up on him, or maybe she wanted more control, I don't know. What did this mean for her husband? That the nurses had to perform all of the routine measures they would normally perform: waking him up to take vital signs, taking his temperature rectally, giving him a liquid medicine that tasted awful. I asked them why and they told me that the wife refused to sign the paperwork. I understand her grief, if that's what it was, but it had a cruel outcome.

എ

Now you know the basics about cancer and what to expect as your friend moves from diagnosis through treatment. It's time to start practicing the many ways in which you can help your friend, following along the course of a typical cancer treatment plan.

CARE ALERT

When your friend is having unrelieved side effects from treatment, remind her to call the doctor. A night spent in pain or nausea will sap her strength, not help her heal.

Chapter Three

Cancer Treatment Options: How to Help

✧

A TYPICAL CANCER treatment path starts with surgery, then chemotherapy, then radiation, then antirecurrence drugs. Your friend's plan may be different for many reasons, so you may find yourself skipping around this schedule.

Surgery and/or Reconstruction

Surgery to remove cancer may be simple or complicated. Same thing with the recovery period. With today's one-minute hospital stays, this can be a time when patient and family really need some help. The patient, for all of his or her suffering, is living with plenty of pain relief. The kids are not.

How to help? Over time, I've changed my mind about hospital visits. I used to think you should rush to the hospital and stay there until your friend checked out. Now I know that your friend is going to need more help at home than in the hospital, so save your energy for that.

There are some big exceptions. If your friend has nobody else, your company is important. If your friend is foggy, he needs an alert friend. If the hospital has a shortage of nurses, he's going to need an advocate who will make sure he is getting the best possible care.

Experienced patients have a few tips for you to pass along to your friend. If possible, she should try to be the first surgery of the surgeon's day. She'll most likely be fasting from the night before, so it's easier because you're not hanging around waiting with nothing to eat or drink. Also, emergencies happen in hospitals and your surgery can easily be delayed by them. This is less likely to happen in the morning. It's not always possible to get the first slot, and it might not be convenient if your friend has a long drive to the hospital. But it's worth a try.

Some patients like to have company while they are waiting to be wheeled away into surgery. This is a job more likely to be given to a spouse or adult child than a friend, but I've seen plenty of friends do it really well. They chat, tell stories, and generally help the patient to relax.

Nobody, not the spouse or the kids or the friends, needs to hold a vigil in the waiting room while your friend is unconscious in surgery, if the surgery is going to be long.

Give the surgeon a cell phone number and go get something to eat. Pick a comfortable restaurant with booths and relax. A vigil in a waiting room chair doesn't help your friend. It just wears you out, like a flight does. Your friend will come out of the recovery room and you're exhausted and just want to go to bed. See the problem? If the surgery is long, skip the vigil.

Chemotherapy

Chemotherapy may last for three months, six months, or longer. Each person has an individual response to chemotherapy; many people have hair loss and fatigue and compromised immune systems, plus the potential for nausea. Chemo can be the most challenging part of treatment.

Let's start with how chemo works. Its goal is to destroy cancer at the cell level. It does this by attacking any cells that are multiplying rapidly, which is what cancer cells do. Chemo can't tell cancer cells from normal ones, so it also attacks healthy but rapidly multiplying cells, such as the ones that grow your hair.

Whether your friend will have other side effects is unknown, but make sure he knows that chemotherapy is not what it is in movies like *Wit, Pieces of April,* and even episodes of *ER.* Today's antinausea drugs, for example, give many patients a barf-free ride. You might not feel so great, but you don't feel seasick.

Some people fear nausea more than they fear cancer. This is real. Relaxation, meditation, medication, exercise, and a little ginger tea can all help. If your friend has a tippy tummy, do him a favor and don't talk about it—and don't tell stories about roller coasters and merry-go-rounds. I think many people fear nausea because they've had three experiences with it: morning sickness, seasickness, and hangover sickness. Chemo nausea has nothing in common with those, because your friend will be given relief before feeling anything. Doctors are going to give him a world of antinausea medicine that will amaze you, and make you want some for yourself (they'll say no).

Fatigue is a common side effect of chemo. It builds up over time. If your friend charted his fatigue, you could see it slowly getting bigger and cycling from pretty good to pretty bad and back again. He might feel it the most a few days after treatment. Rest is a requirement, not an option, of chemo fatigue. If he's not sleeping, he has to talk about it with the doctor.

Mild exercise can help. I used aromatherapy to help, too, meaning that I plugged in some "aroma balls" in the house and in the car's lighter. I used grapefruit oil and spearmint to help me feel more alert. Lavender has the opposite effect; you can replace the little pads in your aroma balls with lavender when you want to rest. You can buy aromatherapy materials at health food stores, but I also like *www.natures gift.com*. Don't use the candle-type aromatherapy diffusers—when you're fatigued and trying to go to sleep, candles are a really bad idea.

The intensity of side effects varies tremendously from person to person. I've seen women without an ounce of vanity become completely panicked at the idea of hair loss. I've seen men who have faced combat be terrified of nausea. I've also seen whiny little complainers rise to the occasion and sail through chemo, inspiring everyone along the way. It's completely unpredictable, and you won't know your friend's reaction until he's well into it.

Some of the medicines they give you to prevent side effects can cause drowsiness, so most chemo sessions will require a driver. This is not the time for your friend to

> **"I loved it when my friend . . . "**
>
> ". . . Sent me her favorite funny book and movie once I was done with the depression of diagnosis. I couldn't believe she liked these things, but that itself gave us a great laugh."
>
> ". . . Helped me to understand appointments and research."
>
> ". . . Set up a *www.lotsahelping hands.com* page for me. We decided that it would be good for my teenager to organize the page so he could feel helpful."
>
> ". . . Dropped off meals. Put them in a cooler and didn't even ring the doorbell while I was asleep."

tough it out. The patient needs a ride to and from, even if he insists on being alone for the treatment itself.

If you or others can't help with driving, let your friend know that there are volunteer organizations that can help.

Ask the treatment center or look at the resources in Appendix A. There can be many reasons why driving the patient would be difficult. If the patient is being treated at a major city center, you may be worried about driving on unfamiliar streets, finding parking, or paying for parking. (Whoever drives the patient, ask about validation parking programs for cancer patients.)

It's usually impossible to predict when an individual chemo session will finish, except it'll almost always be longer than you expect it to be. The doctor may be running late and you will need patience. This is not a department where anybody can rush through their job. The patient before your friend may have had a lot of questions. Your friend might also have a lot of questions, so be tolerant now.

The Chemo Setting

Here's what the setting will probably be like, if you decide to be a chemo buddy.

Because there can be dangerous side effects of chemo, patients are rarely in a private setting (unless it's inpatient treatment). Your friend will be in a large room, with privacy curtains, where he can be seen from a central nurses' station.

Take a walk; you'll see that there are all types of responses to chemo, for patient and buddy alike. I've seen a chemo buddy crying, with the patient comforting her. I've seen an elderly patient stare at her son for three hours, during which he never spoke to her. I've seen patients talk as loudly on their cell phones for an hour as if they were those same annoying people at a great restaurant (they probably were!). One chemo buddy played the cello, choosing mournful dirges so sad that I was ready to take that bow and spank him with it. I've seen husbands and wives looking terrified and unable to help each other yet.

There are many ways to be an effective chemo buddy. The most important quality is the kind of helpfulness that people find easy to accept. "I'm thirsty—what can I get you to drink?" "It's cold in here—would you like a blanket?" "Would you rather take it easy or take a walk?" "They've got magazines—I'll go get a few."

You can also ask the chemotherapy nurse what he or she thinks is most helpful for patients. Ask if they come around with food or if you should go get some for your friend. Some treatment centers have volunteers who bring sandwiches, others don't. You may be surprised to hear that chemo patients can be hungry, but they often get peckish.

Dealing with Chemo Side Effects

Chemo is typically a big challenge but there are many ways to cope, medical and otherwise. You should always encourage your friend to be honest with the medical team about side effects.

I believe that stoicism kills more people than cancer does! It's very important to learn to be realistic about symptoms and side effects. This is not a sign of weakness in your friend, it's a sign of intelligence.

What can you do? When the patient calls you at 9:00 at night and says he's feeling exceptionally dizzy, you get him on the phone to the doctor "on call." There is always a doctor on call in oncology, and they expect to be called for side effects. Remind your friend: If you take care of the symptoms, you feel stronger. If you feel stronger, you'll handle everything better. Dizziness, for example, can be a sign of dehydration. That can make him feel awful, but half an hour after he starts getting some intravenous fluid, he will feel fabulous.

Your job as a friend is to keep reminding him to call. Many, many people don't like calling the doctor. We are convinced that we are bothering them. You can help your friend by encouraging him to get over this. Oncologists need to be called and want to be called.

Some people are just uncomfortable talking about their bodies, even with the doctor. If your friend finds parts of the body to be unmentionable, he's got some work to do. If he's nervous, tell him that I had to tell my dignified, distinguished, revered, and handsome oncologist that I had diaper rash. I'm absolutely serious. If I can make myself tell a doctor that I have diaper rash, your friend is not allowed to keep anything to himself. Especially since the doctor said, "Ouch, that's too bad. It's not a side effect of this treatment, though."

Radiation

Radiation is a painless, invisible treatment for some types of cancer. Radiation differs greatly from cancer to cancer, and can cause a sunburnlike rash, but its main symptom is fatigue, and it can be pretty crushing.

Your friend will have a planning session on a mockup of the real radiation machine. They will mark him with tiny tattoos to help them line up the radiation beams. Sometimes they'll be making a mask to be worn for treatment of the brain.

When radiation starts, it usually means a daily treatment with weekends off. Your friend will lie on a table, and everyone will leave the room as they do when you have an X-ray. The treatment itself takes a minute or two, plus a few minutes to position your friend on the table in exactly the right position. As with any doctor's appointment, there will sometimes be delays, but if all goes well, this is typically a fifteen-minute appointment.

For most people on a standard twenty-eight-day treatment plan, the first two weeks are pretty breezy. After that, the fatigue often sets in. I found that I could manage the fatigue by planning my day around it. If I wanted to go out at night, I had to rest first.

Radiation side effects vary greatly by body part and severity, however. I once had a five-day program that I expected to smile my way through, only to feel seasick and tired. It happened because the radiation penetrated the organs, which it does not usually do with treatment of the breast. So if your friend is having a tough response, be understanding and make sure that the radiation oncologist knows about it. They can help.

At the end of radiation, it can take a few weeks or even months before your friend feels great again. I don't know if it's the radiation or the combination of months of treatment. I've noticed that people who have a lump removed and have radiation, as opposed to major surgery and chemotherapy, recover more quickly. But everybody is different. I love the fatigue advice a postpartum nurse once gave me: Don't take your bathrobe off for two weeks after the baby arrives. Your robe sends a clear signal that you are still recovering. Nobody asks you to do a thing. No visitor expects coffee unless they go in and make it themselves. My husband wants to know if I plan on getting dressed anytime soon, since that baby was born twenty-one years ago.

I think not. It's good advice for some of the days of cancer treatment, too.

How can you best help your friend during radiation? Driving. Company. When I started radiation I decided to go by myself each day. Your friend might do that, and maybe it'll work. For me, the fun wore out in a couple of days. I don't know why, exactly. But I needed company, and I needed to have someone else do the driving. I really treasure the time I spent with all of the special people who volunteered. It made the long radiation weeks pass more quickly, gave me time with friends, and took the stress out of the day. Those are all good things that help you get up and go again tomorrow.

If your friend is trying the lone wolf approach, keep an eye on things and see how it's going. If his method isn't working, you can step in and help. How can you tell it's not working? He sounds depressed about going—or he talks about skipping a treatment day. That's your cue. By the way, even if you go along with your friend, you will not be able to be in the room when the dose of radiation is actually done.

Cancer-Prevention Drug Challenges

Cancer can be a hormone roller coaster for many patients. Chemotherapy may induce menopause, which is sudden.

Many patients begin antihormone therapy also. Antihormone treatments can be breezy for some and very challenging for others.

Antihormone therapy is used if the type of cancer is fed by hormones, such as estrogen or testosterone. Cancer needs to be starved, and these drugs help. When I first started them, everything about them sounded bright and cheery. There would be "mild" side effects, said the drug company Web sites.

Many people have mild side effects, but I did not like the roller coaster of emotions, the hot flashes, the sweats. I had already experienced instant menopause, caused by chemo. That wasn't bad at all, just normal old menopause. This was different. I was a little surprised; I had tolerated chemotherapy and radiation pretty well, and suddenly I felt like I had tripped just before the finish line.

I'm not alone, and your friend may face the same challenge. The well-known secret is that some patients stop taking these drugs. Before your friend does that, he needs to have a completely honest discussion with his oncologist, because they have quite a few ways to help and there are plenty of people working on this problem. The first person to come up with a nonhormone cure for the symptoms of menopause will never have to work again.

Some oncologists are not that focused on treating these side effects, so your friend may have to get help from a doctor who is a gynecologist, an endocrinologist, a urologist, or a psychopharmacologist.

Your friend may need reassurance about seeing a psychopharmacologist. He may think that you think he is crazy, or that his symptoms are psychosomatic. The truth is, nobody knows why psychopharmacological drugs can help with side effects. If they did, they could cure them. Nobody knows exactly how and why a hot flash gets started, for example, so you can guess that nobody knows what can stop one, except hormone replacement therapy, of course, which the oncologist will stress is a bad idea.

There's not a lot you can do to help during this stage except encourage your friend to seek help. Do all of the research you can, but be wary of "natural cures" for symptoms, because they may contain the same ingredients that are in manmade ones. As always, it's important for your friend to review any supplements with the oncologist.

I tried everything, from antidepressants to acupuncture. I keep a fan on all night, aimed near my face. I even tried a tiny dose of belladonna. Nobody believes that I took belladonna, because it sounds like something from an elegant English murder mystery—and it is. It comes from the deadly nightshade plant, and while you can kill your elderly but brutal uncle, the lord of the manor, by mixing it with his port, it can also help with hot flashes. It works for some people, it didn't work for me.

Hypnosis, however, is a tool that can relieve symptoms. It is not a cure, but it definitely helps. If your friend is open to alternative treatments, encourage them to do some research on local hypnotherapists. Or you can take the lead and gather information for them to look over.

Lymphedema

Whenever someone has surgery or radiation to their lymph nodes, there is a possibility that they can develop lymphedema, which is fluid collection in the limb nearest the lymph nodes you had removed. It can be a minor problem or a major one. The most important thing for you to know is that if your friend is having swelling in a limb where she had lymph nodes removed, she should call the doctor. Help her by insisting.

Many cancer patients who develop lymphedema feel that their surgeons do not take it very seriously. That is sometimes true, because oncology surgeons are focused on life-threatening problems and they tend to think of other problems as minor. For your friend the patient, however, lymphedema can be a big deal and you are going to hear a lot about it.

What is it? Lymphedema is basically swelling, or collection of fluid. Lymph fluid is thick. It cannot find the old lymph nodes that used to pump it around the body and so it sits there. It starts to back up like a slow drain. The limb swells, sometimes dramatically.

Why is that a problem? For some women, it's cosmetic. One hand is bigger than the other, one arm is bigger. Rings and bracelets don't fit anymore.

But if the problem worsens, it can be very uncomfortable. Your friend's skin feels tight, or the swollen area feels sensitive. I find that I don't know what size my arm will be throughout the day, so I have given up on tight sleeves. I wear nothing but knits now, big knits. You could fit another person in my sleeves with me, which is not pretty but at least I know my tops will fit all day.

Air travel can worsen lymphedema, so if your friend develops it she should talk with her surgeon before getting on a plane. It can also start at any time after the initial surgery, even years later.

But there is one more problem with lymphedema that isn't about comfort or appearance. Lymph fluid is a wonderful environment for bacteria. If your friend has a lot of lymph fluid sitting around in a spa like her nice warm arm, and even a little bacteria gets in there, she can quickly develop a serious infection. The affected area is much more sensitive to infection than the rest of your body; an unaffected limb can resist infection from a cut much more strongly than one with lymphedema.

How can your friend manage lymphedema? There are massage methods, sleeves, and newly designed pumps that can help. The goal is to get that fluid moving and keep it moving. The massage technique should be done initially by a professional, such as a physical therapist, and taught to the patient. Your friend should also review with her doctor what to do if her condition changes. With the initial swelling, for example, she might see her surgeon or primary doctor, who will probably get her in for lymphatic massage and basic training about living with lymphedema. There may even be a lymphedema clinic in her area specializing in treatment. For more information, see Appendix B.

With future swellings—you hope there will be none, but there can be—she won't necessarily head for the surgeon's office again. She'll do her special massaging, or pumping, or sleeve wearing. However, if the swollen area turns red, your friend may be starting to brew an infection called cellulitis. It's time to call the doctor, and it's usually time to start antibiotic treatment right away. This can be a serious infection, and it will get worse quickly.

> **"I loved it when my friend . . . "**
>
> ". . . Brought meals, stayed and ate with us, cleaned up afterward."
>
> ". . . Took the dog when he was sprayed by a skunk. I don't know how she stood it, but I couldn't do it at that time. She found a groomer who would make him minty fresh again."
>
> ". . . Did errands that couldn't wait, like signing the kids up for sports, returning videotapes and library books, getting the car inspected or the tank filled, taking the dog for a rabies shot."

If your friend's arm is swollen and red and she also develops a fever, it's usually time to head to the emergency room. She's probably going to need intravenous antibiotics and may be staying for a few days.

Your friend can have lymphedema forever without ever developing an infection, of course. Still, there are some general guidelines she can follow to help avoid one. These include: Avoid anything that would expose an affected area to germs; wear gloves while gardening; avoid heavy lifting; don't handle raw meat without gloves; if there's a cut keep it clean and covered; avoid sunburn. Many people will advise your friend not to go for manicures. If she does, she should bring her own set of tools with her. Trimming cuticles is one way to let bacteria in, so if she is going to have her cuticles cut (against advice), make sure she is extra careful about sterility.

You can't cure your friend's lymphedema, but encourage her to have a plan. Here's the protocol my surgeon, Dr. Susan Troyan, mapped out for me.

When the problem developed I worked with a physical therapist trained in lymphatic massage. Then I moved to using a pneumatic pump daily, then tapering to once a week (mine is from NormaTec; it is a big sleeve that does a soothing simulation of the lymphatic system). I add in more pumping sessions if I have done something that might increase my risk of developing an episode of swelling, such as air travel or manicures. Some people wear a compression sleeve for travel. I find even a little bracelet confining, so the sleeve is impossible.

If I develop swelling, I increase the pump use and try to keep my arm elevated higher than my heart. If the arm reddens, I start antibiotics and let the doctor know. If my arm is hot and I spike a fever, I go to the emergency room. If I travel in the United States, I carry a paper prescription that is undated. Overseas, I carry a supply of the antibiotics.

This plan has kept me free of cellulitis since my first and only episode.

∾

That's the typical path of your friend's medical treatment. For some it has started and finished in a month, for others it has gone on for a year, for some it will go on indefinitely. Throughout treatment and beyond it, you and your friend are starting to learn one thing about cancer that stuns everyone new to it: None of us have any idea how to communicate. Good communication is a life-giving practice for a sick friend, while bad communication saps her strength, so we'll cover it in detail next.

Chapter Four

I Know I'll Say the Wrong Thing!

CANCER PATIENTS, LIKE pregnant women and the star of a bachelor party, have one universal experience: They will hear some of the dumbest, most thoughtless comments you can imagine. I know that because I've said all of them. I hate to admit it, but I say a lot of stupid things, like:

Him: My wife is pregnant!
Me: Say goodbye to sex!

Her: I'm getting married!
Me: I hope you like picking up socks!

Him: My mother has melanoma.
Me: My mother died of that!

Her: I have stage III cancer.
Me: They can cure anything nowadays!

Why do we say stupid things? It starts because our brains are divided into friend sections, like a theater or a ballpark. Your best friend has the best seat in the house. If your best friend tells you she has cancer, you're only thinking of her. You won't say anything stupid, because you're too busy listening to her. "I'll be there for you," is what you'll say.

You'll say smart and helpful things to everybody in the good seats in your brain. But as the seats get farther and farther from home plate, or the stage, you start slipping. By the time you reach the last row in the bleachers, that's when your brain drags up everything that very worst aunt of yours always blurted out at family gatherings.

See? When somebody from the back row tells you their news, you barely hear them. Their news just reminds you of events in your life. That's why you tell the newly engaged neighbor that you hope she likes picking up socks. You wouldn't say that to your best friend, not even if her dream man hasn't picked up a sock since he first threw one out of his cradle. Whatever the case and whoever the friend, first things first: Check your mouth and open your ears.

How to Listen

Listening is a well-studied art. There are academic studies, corporate studies, bestselling books, and training programs.

If you search on Google for "trained listening," you'll get zillions of results. If you have worked for a moderately large company, you've probably had to go to a workshop on "*Productive Listening*" or "*Listening for Results.*"

I start with a simpler approach: Are you a dog or a cat? I'm serious. If you don't have either one of these pets, borrow one for the purposes of this little test.

STEP 1
Put the cat on the floor in front of you.
Tell it your life story.

STEP 2
Put the dog in front of you. Tell it your life story.

You already know what happens, don't you? The dog hangs on your every word. He sits with his ears forward, aimed at you, only you. If you sound happy, his tail will wag and he will pant with excitement. If you sound angry he will be very sad. True, he's really just waiting to see if you have any food, but that doesn't matter. You will feel as if he listened carefully. And he did. The cat, if he has not fallen asleep or walked out of the room, is working on hacking up a furball.

So if you want a simple answer to "how can I be a good listener," it's Be A Dog.

You probably don't know yet if you're a good listener or not for your cancer patient friend. For one thing, every patient is different, every friend is different. Your listening style that works really well for you at work may be a disaster for your friend. So let's start by finding out what your listening style is.

Listening Lessons: Take the Personality Test

This is a simple test. Your answer to the questions in the chart (on the facing page) will determine what type of "listening personality" you have.

Let's say your friend who has cancer has just said: *"I am so scared."* What is your first reaction? Take a minute, think honestly. What do you say first? Circle one or more of the answers in the chart, and then read on to see your results.

Number One: Fix-It

If you picked number one, you're a "Fix-It" Listener. No matter what anybody says to you, this is what you hear: "I have a problem. Can you fix it?" You recognize yourself, don't you? People come to you when they're stuck. You know how to take a big problem and break it into its many smaller, more manageable parts, until you have a solution.

1. What exactly is scaring you about this? There must be *something* we can do about that.

2. You have nothing to be afraid of! Think positively! Chin up!

3. Sorry—what did you say?

4. I've learned a thing or two about fear, I'll tell you that. When you've been through everything I've been through, you learn to look fear in the eye and knock it out. That's what you've got to do and I'll tell you how I do it.

5. I know exactly how you feel, because I'm so scared too and I don't know what I'll do if you die. I can't stand seeing you suffer, and I cry myself to sleep every night. Your baldness reminds me of it all the time, and I can't stand seeing you looking so awful. Honestly, I don't know how I'm going to cope (begin sobbing).

6. I can only imagine—tell me more?

This is a really good quality you have and the world needs you very much. The problem is that you heard the wrong thing. Your friend didn't say, "Can you fix my problem?" She said, "I am so scared." It's just like she said "I need a drink" and you handed her a straw instead.

Number Two: Aunt Know-It-All

Well, Auntie, you don't really love listening, do you? It's hard for you. Maybe you can't stand to see somebody else whine. Maybe it reminds you of times when you've whined, but wished you hadn't. Maybe you want people to view you as an inspirational coach.

Here's what your friend heard you say: "Don't bother me with your problems." I know that's not what you meant; I know you meant well. Just like the Fix-It, you heard the wrong thing from your friend. You heard "tell me how to stop these feelings," when what she said was "I am so scared."

Number Three: The Daydreamer

Oh, dear, you haven't heard a thing. Your friend was saying something about cancer, which is all she ever talks about, and now she has stopped talking and is just staring at you. You think she's waiting for you to say something. Yikes! What can you do? Pretend you just didn't hear her. Maybe tell her to speak up.

Does this happen to you often? If it does, you need a little self-training. Start with small doses of listening to a radio station without changing the station. I mean sit down for five minutes, turn on one radio station, and leave it on that no matter what. It doesn't even matter if it's a talk station or music.

Whatever you can do for five minutes, you can do for ten, and fifteen, and more. You love your friend, right? And I'm guessing that you have this daydreaming problem in other parts of your life. If you've ever been in a meeting and been asked your opinion, and you give an opinion about a topic that was voted on twenty minutes ago, you need help. Try the radio exercise until you can do it easily. Then be a Dog for your friend.

Number Four: Mirror, Mirror

You really like to talk. You feel that people like to listen to you, and they probably do. But you're not listening back. Like the others, you heard the wrong words. You heard your friend say "Lecture me about your experiences with fear."

It's very hard to figure out that you're the Mirror-Mirror listener, because you're so comfortable talking. There is an exercise you can do to test yourself: timing. Seriously. There are a few methods. The best is to have someone you trust time you in a group setting. They don't need a stopwatch. They can just silently make little x's on a notepad whenever you're speaking. Some people count "one one thousand, two one thousand," or you just try to make marks at a steady pace.

> **" I loved it when my friend . . . "**
>
> ". . . Took my kids on family trips with them, especially during recovery periods. Sometimes it was camping for a weekend, sometimes it was a day trip to a water park or an evening trip to a pizza place. It helped a lot."
>
> ". . . Did my Remembering—the physical forms that are due at school, the markers and pencils for special projects, replacing all the glue sticks that dried up over the summer."

When someone else speaks, they make little o's. At the end of the event or party or meeting, take a look. There they are—x after x after x. Not so many o's.

You have to learn to pass the mic a little more often. Think of a conversation as a seesaw. You should be going up and down pretty much equally.

Number Five: Bess

Nancy Drew has two really close female friends, George and Bess. George is a brick and can be relied upon in a crisis, such as being kidnapped. George is sporty. Bess's only great quality to have in a friend is that she likes to eat. She's always ready to meet for lunch. With pie. Other than that, Bess is just not a coper. Easily frightened, easily hurt, oh, dear God, you could smack her sometimes. By the way, Bess can be a man or a woman.

How do you figure out if you're a Bess? People are comforting you when their problems are much worse than yours. How do you fix your Bessness? It's hard. You'll have to keep monitoring your speech and catching yourself. You can try the exercise of having a whole conversation without ever referring to yourself. See if you can do it—no saying "I," "me," "my," "myself." If you can do that, there is hope. If not, stay as quiet as you can for as long as you can, so your friend can talk. *Just listen.*

Number Six: The Great Listener

You heard the emotion your friend expressed, not just the words. You've put yourself aside and you're focused on your friend. You're encouraging her to keep going. "Tell me more," you say often. You're leaning forward. You have turned off your cell phone and put down your book.

You even have Great Listener body moves. You make eye contact, except to look up to the heavens and reflect on what she said. If your legs are crossed, they're crossed in the direction of your friend. You're nodding to indicate that you're listening. Not nodding off, smartypants. Your face is expressive—anyone could see what you're feeling. You're engaged in an active conversation of give and take. You could have your own talk show if only you had a friend with a band.

✑

Nobody is a perfect listener. Everybody worries about "saying the wrong thing" to a cancer patient. The only wrong things you can do are to say nothing or to say something without thinking. But still, your worry is real.

Let's start to deflate that worry by understanding it. If you say "the wrong thing" to your friend, what will be the consequences, exactly? She already has cancer, so you're not going to make her sick by saying something. She does know she has cancer, so you're not shocking her by bringing it up. You might hurt her feelings in some way, but surely you've done that before. She'll forgive you. That being said, what should you know to avoid right off the bat?

- Telling somebody else about your friend's cancer when she has asked you not to.
- Talking to her kids about it when she hasn't sat them down yet.
- Saying you'll do something and not doing it.
- Giving her unsolicited advice.
- Giving her solicited advice when you should just say that you don't know the answer.
- Talking nonstop because you can't stand silence.
- Expecting her to want to talk about cancer all the time.

Whatever might slip out despite your best efforts, remember: It's your actions that speak louder, just like Mom said.

Do You Say This? "Call Me If You Need Anything"

The one sentence every caring person says to a cancer patient is "Call me if you need anything." I'm not saying it's a *bad* thing to say. But few cancer patients have ever called, even when deeply in need. Why do patients rarely ask for help, even when they really need it? You want to help, but you'll never, ever be called. Why?

Well, think about your own life. Have you ever called someone and asked for help? Maybe you've called a sibling, or your very best friend, but have you ever called any of your neighbors and other perfectly good friends and asked them for a ride, or an errand, or a meal?

No, because you've been taught to be self-reliant. You teach your kids to be self-reliant. Same goes for the cancer patient. Calling for help requires him to swallow a great big glass of Change. Right now, during this crisis, he just can't do it. Calling a casual friend and asking for help requires more emotional energy than doing a job yourself.

But the physical energy challenge is great, and the patient is going to need help in order to be at his strongest. He needs help! He can't figure that out for himself, and if you can help him learn how, you'll be a major positive part of his healing.

The way you learn to listen now is a big start to teaching your friend to accept your help. You'll need to probe to find out what he needs most. Don't keep telling him you're willing to do whatever he needs. Instead, find out what he needs and get it done. How? In a short visit you can learn a lot. Stacks of takeout boxes tell you some meals would help. An unusually messy house tells you that fatigue is setting in.

The kids can be a good source of information, because they can't hide the fact that they're missing soccer games, or they don't have the supplies they need for a homework project. Kids can have a lot of trouble asking for help, but if you have children in the same class at school, you'll know lots of ways. Take the child with you to buy poster board. Offer rides. Have the kids over for homework sessions. Listen if the child wants to talk. (Don't try to be the child's therapist.) Set up sleepovers.

Try his spouse; his best friend; the kids' teacher; his family. No luck? In the ideal world, you just ask your friend what he needs, he tells you, and you do it. Instead, you'll just have to imagine what anyone would want and try those things out.

Go through a list of your own needs and think about what you would love to have done for you when you have a cold. Maybe you like to keep the car filled with gas so you can always get going? Groceries? Meals? Errands? Laundry? Chores? Lawn care? Making sure the family knows about any sports schedule events or deadlines?

❦

The tips in this chapter will be useful for many situations beyond cancer. I hope it will comfort your friend to know why people say such thoughtless things, to know that she has probably said a few of them herself, and to let go of the tension people might make her feel.

You'll be starting a list of things to try now. But before you just dive right in, you need to gather a bit more information if you're going to really help your friend. You need to have a real sense of what they're going through with their particular cancer, and what exactly it will mean for them in the weeks, months, and years ahead. And it may help you to know that cancer is going to bring out sides of both of you that you've never seen before. On to that discovery next.

CARE ALERT

Should your friend listen to your problems now, too? Yes. Not when she's feeling her worst, of course, but when she's feeling well, start talking. A good friend knows it's your turn.

Chapter Five

How Cancer Brings Out the Best
(and Worst) in Your Friend

❧

YOU DON'T KNOW a friend until you've seen him in a testing crisis. Cancer is one of many testing crises, and everyone shows a different and new side of him- or herself in dealing with it. When the *Titanic* sank, there were the people helping other people; the people praying; the people panicking; the stoics, waiting their turn . . . and maybe even some men dressing up as women to get on those lifeboats.

In movies, it's always the sweetest person who gets sick, of course. It's Beth who dies in *Little Women*, not Jo. I know, we all love Jo, but on the sweetness scale, Beth is at the finish line before Jo has laced up her boots. In real life, our personalities are part Beth, part demon. Cancer doesn't change that. You'll see many qualities in your friend that you haven't seen before, just as you'll see many in yourself.

Watching someone have cancer is like watching sunshine through a glass prism, when you see all of the colors of the rainbow. The cancer prism shows you many different angles of friends. Sometimes you will see all of these on the same day. Sometimes you will like what you see, sometimes not. Your friend may be her steady self through treatment, but is more likely to be as changeable as a teenager. One day she'll be meditating, the next she'll be swearing angrily, the next she'll be weepy. Or she may be all of those in the same hour.

The Spiritual Friend

The spiritual friend may have had a deep faith before cancer, or it may be new. If you are partners in this, it will be an extraordinary experience for both of you. The power of prayer, the power of faith communities, the mystical presence of miracles will move you and transport you. Even if you are not religious, even if you are of a different faith, try going along for the ride with your spiritual friend. An open mind is fresh air for your soul. You can draw the line wherever you are comfortable.

I would guess that nearly every doctor has seen miraculous events. There are people who come back from as close to death as you can get. Very often prayer is involved and invoked. I believe in it. I also believe that if God is being asked to intervene in an illness, He does not always say yes. He often says no. This can be devastating, to feel that God is not on your side. We all know incredibly wonderful people who die far too young. We've all seen miserable people that God kept around for ninety years. We don't know why, and we're not going to find out.

I'm sure I don't have to tell you that spiritual companionship and recruitment are different things. Neither the patient nor the friend should view this illness as an opportunity to get a new member for their faith. It's not nice. I've seen a patient

> **" I loved it when my friend . . . "**
>
> ". . . Gave me a cordless phone with a ringer shut-off, caller ID, and an answering machine."
>
> ". . . Got groceries."
>
> ". . . Took out the trash."
>
> ". . . Told the kids to start taking out the trash. Told them how to do a good job at it."

who was hounded by a neighbor who was convinced that her faith could save him. I've also seen a patient befriend a missionary who dutifully delivered meals and favors, but then the patient refused to go to his church even once.

Also, everyone has different expressions of faith. Some people like a neon faith that everybody can see and share in. Others prefer candlelight. In this case you have to let your friend take the lead. You may pray before every little thing in life, he might not. He may be appalled that you pick up a fork without saying grace, you may be shocked that he doesn't know the Our Father or the Schma. Let him decide what he would like. Ask if he would like you to lead a prayer, don't simply start one.

Faith and the Doctor's Office

What about mixing faith with your doctor and hospital? It can be a great gift to arrange for a visit from clergy if the patient is craving it. You can call a house of worship that is not your own, where you don't know anybody, and still ask them if someone can visit your friend for whatever spiritual reason. Very few clergy would say no to that.

Many people are nervous calling a religion they are not part of. If this is how you feel, remember that you are doing this for your friend. And seriously, I've never come across a religion that did not welcome others or that turned away somebody's need.

Captain Courageous

There are people who stride into cancer with their heads held high. I wasn't one of them. I was irritated that there were so many heroes with cancer. I couldn't stand watching the Olympics because every athlete seemed to have overcome cancer. Everybody told me about heroes, heroes, and more heroes. I knew I had nothing in common with them.

But your friend may be just such a hero, because it turns out that a lot of cancer patients are. They weren't that way when they started, but they got that way real fast. It doesn't take deep courage to start treatment—well, not lots of it, anyway. *It takes courage to keep going back.* If your friend is courageous, you're going to be inspired by this experience and even learn a few things. (Though don't tell your friend that God's plan was for him to get cancer so that you could learn courage.)

Be sure to make room for days when his courage is failing him. Nobody gets through cancer without any moments or even days and weeks of anxiety or even misery. Just be sure to keep reminding him of the courage he has displayed and how he inspires you and everyone else. There's something about being told you have courage that makes you believe that you do.

The Comedian

There are people who are party people. They love to laugh, they love company, and they might sustain that through cancer. I believe strongly in laughter as a stress-releasing, restorative, and healing force. In theory, everybody agrees with me. In actual practice, people get mighty huffy about cancer and they don't want to hear any laughter. If your friend is a laugher, somebody is going to accuse her of being in denial. Tell her not to listen. She's got a great tool in her toolbox. Are you the funny friend? If you can make your friend laugh, you're giving her a gift. You'll laugh together in the chemo area, and your laughter will travel to other patients. You may get frowns from people, including doctors and nurses, who feel you're not behaving appropriately. As a funny person, you know there is only one thing for you to do: Make fun of them. Seriously. Just close the curtain first.

There are no funny cancer jokes, but some people can be very funny about side effects. If I were you, I would leave it to the patient to take the first step on that front. I loved hearing people's clever ideas about what might be done with a bald head—paint a bottom on it. Paint a face and wear your clothes backward. Wear wigs in holiday colors. But again, your best friend might not think being bald is as funny as you do, so let her make the first attempt at humor.

Any kind of humor that makes your friend laugh is good. A book, a movie, a story, a group of friends, a silly magazine. If you laugh together, you'll both feel great.

Chicken Little

Oh, Lord. He screams when an elevator hesitates. His children wear bike helmets when they're sitting on the floor. Does he have a cough? It's cancer! Is he thirsty? It's diabetes!

I know this person well because that's who I am, a complete chicken. I cannot walk on icy sidewalks or wet floors.

I freeze in fear. I must be helped by at least two very strong people. Cancer is either going to help this friend to cope with fear or make him a whole lot worse. A hypochondriac who actually has cancer is a difficult companion. His epitaph will read, "I told you I was sick."

You've got some decisions to make about this friend. If he's stuck in fear, life with him is going to feel mighty long. For one thing, some cancer patients will have new lumps over the years, long after the initial treatment has ended. Just like precancer days, these lumps will probably turn out to be nothing. If he panics over each new lump, are you going to drop everything to sit by his side? Well, yes—but just once. Everyone is entitled to one case of total panic over a new lump or symptom. If he needs more than that, he must call a different friend each time.

I handled my first posttreatment lump really well. I was calm, I put it out of my mind. I was feeling very superior about this, so God, as usual, taught me a lesson. I received a second new lump, and I panicked beyond any reasonable standard of sanity. My husband was away; my sister and her partner entertained me until it was over. My sister even came to the biopsy appointment with me.

You can encourage Chicken Little to reach down deep for a little courage, for the sake of everyone around him. You can remind him that he has handled so much so well. You can encourage him to learn relaxation techniques like meditation and measured breathing. Once upon a time, relaxation techniques meant you would lean back, put your feet up, light a cigarette and make yourself a beverage heavily influenced by gin—but alas, no more. Think yoga instead.

Cancer is an opportunity to tap a kind of courage your friend didn't know she had. It can do the same for you. I believe it's like a muscle that strengthens for you as you need it. It's similar to adrenalin, which gives you a burst of power in an emergency, but this muscle comes to life for long-term challenges—cancer, loss, grief. (You can read more about this in my book, *The Courage Muscle: A Chicken's Guide to Living with Breast Cancer*. All of my proceeds go to a program for cancer patients at Beth Israel Deaconess Medical Center in Boston.)

The New Ager

No friend is less fun than a New Ager. Sorry. I have deep respect for the mind-body connection in other ways; it's just that New Agers spend a lot of time on the floor. They do yoga, Pilates, and meditation, all on the floor. The last time I sat on the floor was in 1997, with one of my children, and it took a crane to get me up. My knees didn't work right for another decade or so.

If your friend was a New Ager before cancer, maybe you have the same interests. Or maybe you've already worked out how to handle your differences. If this is new, though, it's going to be more difficult if you don't share his enthusiasm. He'll want to go to workshops, holistic weekends, labyrinth walking. A labyrinth is usually a flat spiral on the ground, not a maze. You walk the spiral to the center. If you understand the labyrinth idea, this is renewing and relaxing. If you don't, well, keep your thoughts to yourself. Don't ask why someone would walk in a spiral when they could reach the center in three steps if they took a straight line. Don't.

Many of the techniques that we think of as "New Age" are useful tools. Meditation, breathing techniques, and yoga all relieve some of the physical side effects of stress. Stress can hamper the body's ability to heal, so many use these techniques during treatment and beyond, with great results.

You'll have to decide if you want to share in these activities and philosophies. An open mind is a gift you can give your friend, though, so consider keeping him company when he goes to classes.

The Athlete

The number of marathon runners who have had cancer is inspiring and amazing. The ability to run a marathon is incredibly rare among healthy people, and I am in awe of anyone who does it. Just be sure that your friend, whether running a marathon, a triathlon, or playing in a pickup game with seven-foot twenty-year-olds, has talked with his doctor first. Sometimes a little time is needed between treatment and strenuous exercise.

If his athletic goal has been medically cleared, don't stand in the way no matter how scared you are for him.

How could any doctor approve this? That's what you want to say. But if he's healthy enough to do it, and wants to, help out if you can. For example, with your marathoner, arrange a few people who will be at milestones along the way and tell him which ones you'll be at. Cheer him on as he goes by. Have everyone carry a cell phone to keep in touch. Ask him to wear a shirt you can spot in a crowd, because only the winners are running alone. Everybody else is in a big pack. Unless he ends up walking the whole way, in which case he won't be lost in the crowd. But by then it will be dark out.

The Hermit

It's painful to love a hermit who has cancer. You're desperate to help. You're worried beyond belief. You can see that he's pale, or thin, or walking slowly. But he doesn't answer the phone and asks everyone not to drop by. He has no family nearby that you know of.

Most cancer books will tell you that you have to respect people's privacy. In general, cancer patients should maintain the right to go through cancer in their own way. I mostly agree with that, but not always. If your instinct is telling you that the person is lonely and afraid, but ashamed to admit it, then I say ring that doorbell and offer him a ride.

There are also hermits who are surrounded by people. Every office has one. This is the person who didn't even tell anybody she had cancer until she had to, who didn't invite anybody from the office to her wedding. Still look for ways to help her. Tread lightly with the hermit, but still tread!

The Sponge

Lord, keep us from the sponge who has cancer. Make an honest assessment of your sponge friend who has cancer, no matter how much you like him as a friend or his kids, before you go rushing in to help. Before cancer, was your friend the type who always asked for rides to soccer practice but never offered any? Did you take his child on vacation, but your child has never been invited for a sleepover? Did you take care of his sick child while he was at work, and he never said thanks?

Cancer is unlikely to make this person better and highly likely to make him worse. So be careful. You already know if you are vulnerable to this kind of person, and you could become quickly overwhelmed. You and your family must remain more important to you than anybody else. If you have actually volunteered to be a room parent at your child's school more than twice, be on your guard.

Remember, you are trying to help a person in a challenging situation to lead as normal a life as possible. You are not trying to create an invalid who cannot lift his head from the pillow. Providing an unhealthy level of help is like putting a cast on a leg that's not broken: The muscles will atrophy.

It probably sounds cruel to describe any cancer patient as a sponge. But cancer does not turn us into saints, nor does it erase our worst qualities. If you know a sponge, just be cautious about how much you do. And quit reading this book. The last thing in the world you need is to be even more helpful.

The "I Give Up" Friend

One dirty secret of cancer is the number of people who don't do the treatment. They might do the surgery, or a little chemo, but then they quit.

Horrified? Well, let's start by sorting people into sensible groups. If your dad is eighty-seven and is diagnosed with prostate cancer, and he decides against treatment, that's not suicide by cancer. It's common sense. The cancer may or may not kill him, but the treatment might make life mighty unpleasant. In his shoes, you might decline treatment too. But as his child, you want him to live forever. You will push and push. Lots of good fathers and husbands do treatment to make somebody else happy.

Instead of letting your desperate inner child push your parents into treatment, listen to their doctors and listen to Mom and Dad. It's not fair to make somebody live through years of misery, no matter how hard it's going to be for you to accept defeat. They are the only ones who get to decide whether they will take the chance on treatment or not.

> **"I loved it when my friend . . ."**
>
> ". . . Gave me a padded lap desk and a backrest."
>
> ". . . Did 'heavy lifting' chores, like getting out the snow tires, when I was recovering from surgery."
>
> ". . . Took up a collection for a snowplow service and a house cleaning."
>
> ". . . Gave me a super soft, easy-to-put-on top after my mastectomy. It was great during recovery."

Group two is people who can't tough out the treatment. There are plenty of people who are supposed to be taking antihormone drugs, such as tamoxifen or Lupron, but they've stopped. They can't stand the side effects. Plenty of people have no side effects, but many people have hot flashes worse than a sauna in Alabama.

The best way to help this person is with knowledge and with being a buddy for doctor's appointments. You can research and ask questions like: How important is this treatment for your friend's survival? If it makes a major difference, what are all of the methods of reducing side effects? If it makes little difference in survival rates, how much life quality should be sacrificed? The final decision is the patient's, but support from you can be very helpful. Be careful about research and be sure the doctor reviews everything.

The third group has tried everything and is still close to major organ failure. You want to believe that it can be beaten, but his body is shutting down. You're desperate to find the answer that will save him. Every friend needs someone like you, someone who never gives up, someone who is on the phone to a witch doctor in ancient Babylonia who might have a cure. But when the time has come, the only thing that matters is comfort and love. Pain relief, oxygen, room temperature, a gentle foot massage, and a few prayers will make those precious final days wonderful. You won't feel that way in the moment, but you will later.

Now the hardest group: Your friend is sixty. He could live another twenty years with treatment, but decides to stop. His family is desperate and angry. He will say things like "I'm tired of this treatment crap. I've done enough. Life's not worth living if it's going to be like this."

The key message he's giving you is "Life's not worth living." When you know that life is worth living, you will put up with anything that will give you more time. If you feel that your life has value, you will protect it no matter what. But when you forget that, it's hard to get out of bed.

I really believe that this person is usually suffering from fatigue and depression, which are twins. Add loneliness or bitterness and you have a complete family of quadruplets. What do you do? Put cancer aside for a moment. Focus on fatigue and depression to help this friend. See a doctor about it, see a support group, go to a wellness center—do anything you can to find a way to remind your friend that his life is worth living. He's too young for this. It's obviously not your fault if he quits treatment no matter what you do. Just focus on the root causes of the fatigue and depression to help him.

You can't cajole or force somebody into loving life again. But here's one secret: Most people, even when they think life is over, will still do something to help someone else. Ask him to go to an appointment as a favor to you. Ask him to do a little treatment for the sake of his grandchildren. You're appealing to the good person within him and doing him a favor by asking him for help.

Yes, this is guilt-tripping. The baby boomer generation tried to get rid of guilt-tripping. They did not know that it is the major source of maternal recreation during the teenage years. They were wrong. Go ahead.

The Smoker

It is a well known fact among people who work with cancer patients: Many patients do not quit smoking. To the nonsmoker this sounds crazy, but smokers and ex-smokers are nodding their heads in understanding. Because quitting smoking is so difficult, it can be hard to do while under the stress of a diagnosis. For some, the cancer diagnosis is the signal that motivates them. For others, it just can't be beat.

It is hard not to judge a smoker. If you can help someone to quit by taking them to a program, or helping them with support, great. Otherwise, you may just need to stand by and deal with your own pain that your friend won't stop. Nobody can blame you if you can't do it and decide that you need to be the invisible friend (see Chapter 6).

Be sure your friend knows all of the treatments that are available to help with nicotine withdrawal. While the ultimate job of quitting still requires tremendous strength and optimism, there really are some medications that can help to take the edge off.

The Walk-A-Thoner

Many cancer patients become active in fundraising for cancer research, which often involves walk-a-thons. If you believe in a cause and believe in walking for it, join him in the walks or write a check. If you don't, don't. Over your lifetime, you are going to know many people who walk and raise money. You have to decide how much you're going to give each year and to what. Yes, everybody has an obligation to make the world a better place. Not everybody makes the same choices.

If your friend is determined to walk, and you are equally determined not to, this can be a source of friction. Good friends should understand each other's preferences and freedom to choose.

For happy friendships, the amount of money and effort that you give to each other's causes should even out eventually. If I give $50 for your walk, I kind of expect you to buy raffle tickets from my kids. I also put your name on my list of people to ask for money for my favorite causes. I've seen enough friendships get bumpy over this to believe that the smoothest road is a two-way street.

The Achiever

I suppose, if I were Lance Armstrong's friend, I would have told him to take it easy. "Take a break," I would have said. "Pamper yourself, take care of *you*." He would not have heard me, since I would be sitting in a recliner ten miles behind his dust. For Lance Armstrong, my advice would have been stupid. For many people, it's right.

The problem for the achiever is that nobody—including inspirational Lance—makes it through cancer without some fatigue. You can spot a crash-and-burn cancer patient ten minutes after diagnosis. They seem to be going into battle, they will still go to work every day and carpool the kids and learn mountain climbing. While striving is important for all patients, your friend who always does too much is still going to do too much.

You can try to ease him into some new thinking. You can ask him what he's going to take off his plate. He will probably not listen until he finds himself sound asleep in a scanner and begins to think that maybe he could use a little rest.

∽

Now you've gotten to know the many sides of your remarkable "new" friend. One day you'll laugh about it together. To your amazement, he'll say that she felt the same way about *you*.

Chapter Six

How Cancer Brings Out the Best (and Worst) in You

♐♥

CANCER SHOWS YOU many different sides of the patient and many different sides of yourself. You want to be a great friend, and you probably are, or you wouldn't be reading a book about how to help. But just as cancer shows new angles of your friend's personality, it's going to show you a thing or two about yourself. Sometimes you'll be a good friend and sometimes not. Just like the patient, you'll have good days and not-so-good.

Along the way I've discovered quite a few new personality traits, in me and in others. I've been a very good friend, a really awful friend, and a totally crazy one. If you recognize yourself among the people described here, have a good laugh about it and try again tomorrow.

The "You Have Cancer? Dear God, Why Did This Happen to Me?" Friend

You go running to everyone you know—to talk about the burden you are carrying because your friend has cancer. If you took one of those stress quizzes from a magazine, her cancer would go on the list as your biggest problem.

Does this sound familiar? If you recognize yourself, but only occasionally, don't worry about it. There *is* an emotional burden on friends and family when a loved one has cancer, and it's perfectly fine for you to talk about it.

But is this how you are all the time? Are your most serious problems actually other people's problems? Hmm. It's possible that you are a saint, because you're always thinking of others first. Odds are you're not, though. Odds are you don't have a whole lot of heavy burdens to carry on your own, so you are stressed just by knowing somebody who is stressed.

> **" I loved it when my friend . . . "**
>
> ". . . Never questioned my decision about reconstruction."
>
> ". . . Asked me to walk her through my decision on reconstruction so that she could understand it. As I said it out loud, I knew I was doing the right (or wrong) thing for me."
>
> ". . . Walked my dog when I couldn't."

This is a hard personality trait to fix, though life has a way of fixing it for you by handing you a few burdens of your own along the way. In the meantime, keep reminding yourself: "Cancer is not actually happening to me. I need to be strong for my friend while it happens to her."

The "Just Do as I Say" Friend

Did your siblings call you "Know-it-all" as a child?

You looked on the Internet for many hours. You researched your friend's cancer and you feel you know all about it. You've looked up clinical trials all over the world. You tell the patient that her doctors are incompetent, that she needs this treatment or that, that she needs surgery or not. You are insistent that everyone try your alternative treatments or the vitamins you happen to sell.

Or you should be a research doctor, because you are determined to find out what caused her cancer. "When was your last physical?" you ask. Your last PSA test? Your last self-exam? What do you eat? Do you have a family history? Have you tested for radon? Is there asbestos in your basement? Is your town polluted? Do you use deodorant? Do you exercise? Did you ever smoke? Do you fertilize your lawn? Put salt on your sidewalks? Are you now or have you ever been a member of the Communist party?

Cancer patients mostly can't stand this questioning. It implies that something could have prevented this crisis. Maybe it could have. That doesn't help now. It's guaranteed to be upsetting for the patient, so do your best to leave Sherlock Holmes at home.

Do you recognize yourself in this description? You might be undermining your friend's confidence in her treatment or herself. If you feel that your knowledge is important and helpful, ask if your friend would like you to go to a doctor's appointment to help her ask questions. If she says, "No thanks," don't press it.

The best thing you can do for your friend is review your listening skills, and then try this technique: If you have advice to give, say it only once. No cheating: Once.

The Eternal Optimist Friend

I love *Pollyanna*; I love the book and any movie anybody ever wants to make about it. Pollyanna is the persistent—and sorely tested—optimist. When someone has cancer, a little Pollyanna in a friend is a good thing. Here's the risk: There is a fine line between being optimistic and being dismissive of the patient's worries. The friend who says, "You can do this, I know you can, and we'll all be with you" is Pollyanna. The friend who says, "It will all work out for the best so stop worrying," when all you said was that chemo doesn't look like much fun, that's not Pollyanna. That's Pollyanna's evil, dismissive twin.

It is true that a positive attitude helps you to cope with treatment. I don't believe it cures cancer, but I believe it keeps you striving and living well while your body fights it. Your friend is going to be lectured on the importance of a positive attitude by some of the most negative people you both know. Don't be one of them. Just help your friend to laugh about these lectures. My personal favorite pep talk came from the town whiner whose sole cancer experience was thinking she might have had a lump but didn't.

The Herbal Friend

You will not rest until you have the patient eating dirt. Good nutrition is important, of course. But your cancer friend may or may not want to make major lifestyle changes, however important you know that to be for her present and future health. It will be difficult to watch her eat fried lard, but she gets to choose. Offer your expertise, but let her decide whether she wants to hear it or not.

You may have thought I meant something else by "herbal." You probably already know that some cancer patients prefer marijuana for pain management. When I was going through treatment nobody offered me any, and as far as I can tell there are plenty of other legal ways to relieve pain. If your friend asks you to find some for her, you can Just Say No if you want to. Or, suggest that she discuss the matter with her doctor.

The "Oh, That Reminds Me" Friend

Your friend mentions he feels nauseous; you talk about your morning sickness until he is turning greener by the minute. He talks about nerve pain; you talk about shingles. He talks

about hair loss, you talk about the drudgery of shaving. Is this you? Yes, because this is *everybody*. We all do it. Watch yourself over the next few days and see how often you say, "That reminds me" when someone else is talking.

The cure? Try to listen without responding with an anecdote of your own. It's hard, because many of us make conversation that way. It takes practice. To work on this,

> **"I loved it when my friend . . . "**
>
> ". . . Threw me a little head-shaving party."
>
> ". . . Shaved my head quietly, privately, not telling anybody."
>
> ". . . Organized an e-mail list of everyone we know so I could communicate easily."
>
> ". . . Sent me a funny card every week."
>
> ". . . Looked at my new boobs and ooohed."

start by increasing your awareness. Tell yourself you're going to make a note every time you say "that reminds me." Or ask a very close friend, someone you really trust, to do it with you. Make a note "TRM" on a pad for a day for each other or, under the right circumstances, you can even text it!

The Invisible Friend

"I don't know what to say. I get so nervous around medical stuff. I know I'll say the wrong thing."

Every cancer patient has the friend you never hear from. I've been that friend. So has the cancer patient.

Some invisible friends are really just feeling awkward. If that sounds like you, all you need is to decide on your opening sentence. Try any combination of these:

- "I don't know what to say but I want to talk with you because I'm thinking about you all the time."
- "You have a lot of people who care about you and I'm one of them."
- "I heard your news and I wanted to talk and see how you are and if you have any more details now."
- "Can you have chocolate?"

You really can't go wrong if you care about your friend and want to help. If that feeling is sincere and shines through, it doesn't matter what you say.

The truth is, many invisible friends have something else going on, not awkwardness. Does that sound like you? Maybe your friend's cancer is reminding you of someone else's and you can't stand to go through those emotions again. Maybe you're overwhelmed by your own life, justifiably or not, and can't reach out to anybody else. Or, you actually don't understand what the patient is going through. This happens often with younger people—they know little about cancer and have little experience with it. Your friend might be surprised and hurt to find that otherwise loving nieces and nephews don't even send a card. Remind her that they just might not know any better. If you know those kids, let them know that your friend needs to hear from them.

Sometimes the invisible friend did not know what to say at the beginning and avoided the patient. Now, the guilt has snowballed until you think you have to avoid your friend forever. If you recognize yourself as the invisible friend, take action today. Call. Write. Visit. Apologize—briefly. Explain—briefly. Reconnect. Is there a time limit? No. Get in touch.

Do your friend a favor, though, and remember that this is not about you. Don't expect her to listen to a half hour of why you didn't get in touch. Don't keep asking for her forgiveness. Just get in touch and start helping out.

People often tell me how guilty they feel about a friend who has died and so it's too late to do anything. They often ask me to help them to feel less guilty, which you should never ask an Irish Catholic person, because we will just make you feel worse. I can only tell you to learn from this experience and never do it again. Be determined to help your friends no matter how awkward you feel.

The Horror Story Friend

No woman of childbearing age can be frightened by a scary story or a horror movie. It's because we have all been—prepare yourself—to baby showers. Baby showers have been scientifically proven to be the anthropological source of humankind's most frightening legends. See, when a woman announces that she is with child, someone yells "Ladies, Start Your Stories." And they're off! The aunt who died in childbirth, the labor that lasted seven days, the neighbor who lost her mother and father on the day she gave birth to twins.

Cancer is exactly the same. If you like to tell horror stories, you've probably got plenty of cancer stories saved up. You could go on for hours. The cousin who was dead a week after diagnosis. The neighbor who threw up every day of treatment. The friend with the botched reconstruction.

Nobody knows why you think this is helpful, but you do. I'm not accusing you of being mean. I'm just begging you to stop. And move to Hollywood.

The Uber-Boss Friend

It's very hard to recognize this friend in yourself. Try these questions: Do you have a really hard time finding or keeping volunteers to work on your projects? Do you find that people grow silent when you chair a meeting to organize something? Do you know the best way to do everything and life would be so much more efficient if people would do it your way the first time you ask them to?

You're probably smart, talented, and organized, but you've got no patience. You might get away with that at work, but you won't in the cancer setting. People are upset, or worried, or vulnerable, or weepy, and your "take no prisoners" style will not help.

My honest advice? Let someone else take charge. Do the tasks assigned to you and don't keep complaining about how it is being organized. Seriously: Fire yourself, or be the buddy who helps with the insurance company.

The New Friend

Are you a new friend? Every cancer patient has a wonderful surprise in store: People they barely know will come forward in helpful and caring ways. While it's true that some close friends become invisible, twice as often there will be new people in the picture. I don't know why it's true, but it happens to everybody. Sometimes this will be a temporary friendship; others will last a lifetime.

Typically, when you become a new friend to someone with cancer, she has always seemed interesting to you but you never got around to getting together much. In other cases you notice that she has few family and friends nearby. You can start with a phone call asking if you can give her a ride to treatments. You might drop by her house with a basket of food for the kids. You might send a card or an e-mail. You might contact the "head organizer" who is arranging meals. If you are becoming a new friend to someone who already has old friends, I hope the old friends will welcome you into this circle of people who love the patient. They usually will take you in with wide-open arms, but it doesn't always happen that way. I've seen a situation in which the "best friend" of the patient was not organizing any help. The "new friends" decided to step in. The "best friend" got itchy about it—but the patient was grateful and has maintained her new friendships and helped them out when needed, too.

Just keep doing what you want to do to help and keep your focus on the patient. The old friends may come around, or they might not, but you will have helped where it is needed. Be sure to be listening carefully, because as a newcomer, you may not recognize signs of overdoing it or fatigue.

☙

You've learned what you need to know about cancer—the timeline, listening, and understanding yourself, your friend, and your friendship. You're ready for the Toolboxes now.

Chapter Seven

The Toolbox of Practical Ways to Help Your Friend Cope

🌿

YOU'VE LISTENED, YOU'VE prayed, you've given solace. Now your friend is facing the physical challenges of cancer treatment. It's time to take out the toolboxes of practical ideas. But before we get into the first toolbox, let's start with a general tip on how to help—and have your help accepted. Asking for help can be hard for your friend, so to get the ball rolling—make it easy!

The Two-Choice Tip

You have a list of ideas, which you've developed by listening, asking your friend about her needs, and reading through the ideas in this book. How do you get your help accepted? How do you avoid the "Call me if you need anything" trap?

Here's the trick. It's an old sales technique that has been used on you a thousand times: You give the customer a choice between two positive choices. Remember when you bought a car, and the car salesperson asked, which is your favorite color, the blue or the silver? You said silver, and I bet you ended up buying that car. That's the technique. It distracts you from the big question.

Here's how it works. You say: I'd like to take the kids out—would Saturday or Sunday be better? I'd like to go to the kid's soccer games and cheer them on—this weekend or next? Do you want dinner brought tonight or tomorrow night, which is better? I'll visit your Mom at the nursing home for you—can I bring her food or not?

If your friend is religious, offer to drive or walk to services. You'll say, "Would 9:00 or 10:00 be better?" Say your prayers and mean it. Sign him up for prayer groups—meaning that you enter his name.

If he's a shy person, or just overwhelmed and terrified, offer to be a buddy for doctor appointments so that someone will ask questions. You can say "I'd like to take you to a doctor's appointment if you think that would be helpful. When is your next one?"

This chapter will give you specific ideas. In the meantime, if he's depressed, give him the chance to talk freely without making him feel guilty that he can't just snap out of it. If he's a neat freak, take his car and clean it. Or clean the house. If the lawn is looking long, let him know you're going to mow it. If snow comes, talk with him about what he wants to do. If you're a heart-attack-waiting-to-happen, don't volunteer to shovel. That's what teenagers are for.

Make sure that your ideas help this individual patient and are not just what you would want. You might want a day of massage and sauna, the patient might hate that. He might prefer a short walk. You might find swimming the most restorative activity; he might find it chilling. This is hard to understand, especially if you're a great big old bossy person. You just know that you could cure this patient if only he'd come to your spinning class. Meditation would let him breeze through surgery—you just know it. Pomegranate juice is delicious, if only he would drink it! Step back and remember to listen. Try your best to know the difference between encouragement and bossing.

Now, on to ways you can help your friend!

Food

Food is the most basic need, right? We need to start there. So you make your best casserole in your grandmother's special dish and head for your friend's house. It makes you feel very 1950s. You arrive at the house and wonder why there are so many cars. Then you see the parade of casseroles marching up the front walk. Two things are true: Your casserole will never be eaten and you will never see your grandmother's dish again.

Ah, you think. I will volunteer to organize all of these meals and volunteers so that this won't happen. This is a sign that you're young, very young. You'll run into the person who never does what they say they will do, so you end up doing double duty. You'll find the person who doesn't seem to read instructions and puts peanut butter cookies in the bag when the youngest is allergic to peanuts.

Still, it's a wonderful thing to organize meals for a family coping with cancer. Here's how to do it: Start by figuring out what your friend needs. A week of meals? A month of twice-a-week meals? Talk to your friend and her family to get a general sense of what they like and don't like, or if there are any allergies. If they eat a special diet, have a thorough talk. If they're vegetarian, do they eat eggs and dairy? Do they have any favorite ingredients or any that they don't like at all?

Follow some commonsense rules—you don't send foods that contain ham, bacon, or pork to families who are Muslim or Jewish, and you don't send beef to Hindus. There are plenty of exceptions, but these are some general rules to follow that will hopefully spark further questions and thoughts.

Don't let anybody send a container that must be returned. Encourage people to bake in foil containers that you leave there. Pack napkins, drinks, plastic cups, and utensils if you can. This is ecologically incorrect, but it's awfully helpful.

Keep a list, with addresses, so that the family can send thank-you notes. Yes, each person who dropped off a meal should receive a note! Cancer can build community around the patient, but the patient's gratitude is essential for that to last.

Next decide how you're going to organize the organization. Most

> **" I loved it when my friend . . . "**
>
> ". . . Took the kids to church, any church!"
>
> ". . . Mowed the lawn."
>
> ". . . Taught my kids how to mow the lawn and reminded them to do it."
>
> ". . . Helped me in the hospital when I couldn't advocate for myself."

people do a chart of weeks and have people sign up. By week two, if you do this alone, you'll hate the whole world. People, unfortunately, are unreliable. They promise to make dinner, they forget. So you have to remind them. You call. They don't return your call, so you don't know if they're going to do it or not. You find yourself feeding your kids cereal for dinner because you're spending so much time feeding someone else's kids. If you have a high-maintenance volunteer who needs constant reminders, take them off the list. Seriously. They won't even notice.

You need a backup organizer, so that you can do one week at a time and then pass the baton. Some hospitals even offer a Web site where you can set up a schedule and everyone can sign up for what they want to do. It's a good idea for people to say what they're making; even the most grateful friend can eat a roast chicken from the supermarket no more than a couple of times a week.

Set some guidelines about the delivery. Someone recovering from surgery who is alone cannot get down the stairs while a volunteer is ringing the doorbell. Set a delivery time in advance so that the family knows when someone needs to be home to receive meals. Consider placing a cooler at the door so that helpers can drop food off there. Be sure that everyone knows that meals should be finished and just need heating up. Any complicated meal that's going to require more than a minute of work is not very helpful.

Some patients like it when the person who made dinner stays and eats with the family. Most people don't, and most volunteers want to get home, but if company is a big need for your friend or her family, see if some of your volunteers would like to stay.

Here's an odd thing that's helpful to know: Some patients get overwhelmed by the amount of food in the house. Seriously, it actually upsets them. They're unable to throw out "perfectly good food," and there is no more room in the fridge. Scale back the meal delivery if this is really happening, but be sure you get your information from the right family member. I once brought a big meal to a family, but the patient met me at the door and said she wasn't hungry so please don't leave it because smells were bothering her. I had to tell her, "Sorry, this is for your family—they're hungry!" I wasn't my most tactful here, and she doesn't like me anymore (but her kids do). Anyway, find the right way to address everyone's needs as best you can, and be mindful of my mistakes (sending bread during Passover, thinking that vegetarians eat fish, forgetting to write on the bags that there was ice cream to be put in the freezer). Here are some helpful sites to visit:

www.lotsahelpinghands.com
This Web site is a great organizing tool. It lets you set up a calendar that friends and family can use to sign up to help. It's often linked to other Web sites, such as hospitals and groups like Y-ME, but you can also use this link to get there yourself.

www.letsdish.com
This operates in many states. You go and cook in a big kitchen where you can make a million servings of meals,

or they'll do it for you. You freeze lots of meals. Okay, I don't think cooking is fun so I've never actually done this, but my friend highly recommends it. If you have limited kitchen facilities or if you're looking for an activity that will get the coworkers together to do something for the patient, this can be great.

Before you go to Web sites, ask your patient friend if there are cookbooks her family especially likes. If her family is generally trying to eat healthy food, try *The Healthy Family Cookbook* by Dr. Hope Ricciotti and Vincent Connelly. If you want to bring food recommended by cancer experts, try *www.cancerbackup.org.uk/resourcessupport/eating well*; the Recipe Corner at the American Institute for Cancer research at *www.aicr.org*; or *www.cancer.stanfordhospital.com/forPatients/services/nutrition/recipes*. But remember that communication with the family is always the most important key to a successful meal-organizing plan. You may feel that you have to supply "cancer-fighting" foods, while the family may beg you not to! (One of the best cancer sites in the world recommends a sauce made from bran, apples, and prunes, which I believe is an evil thing to give most families with small children.)

Casseroles are the easiest thing to bring; use a foil baking pan. You can search for casseroles at *www.allrecipes.com* or at any of your favorite recipe sites. A casserole on its own is great, but it's even better with a salad and rolls that you buy already made.

Be the Note-Taking Doctor Buddy

All cancer patients are deaf. They cannot remember any details from their meetings with oncologists, especially that first meeting. Luckily my husband heard everything. I don't have a good mind for medicine, so I didn't go to any information appointments by myself. I've gone alone to scans, biopsies, treatments, plenty of other things, but not important information sessions. If, like most people, your friend is no good at doctor's appointments, this is the time when she has to do something about that. She doesn't have chicken pox, she's got cancer, and she has to be paying attention. If she can't or won't, you've got to make sure she brings a buddy with her.

Make sure she chooses her buddy carefully. When she asks them to recap the appointment for her and they're whistling the last song they heard on the radio, you know she'll need a new buddy.

Some people are just plain afraid of doctors. They get nervous, their blood pressure goes up, they don't want to ask any questions. It's time to grow up, but if they can't, you can help. As the doctor buddy, be familiar with the basic issues of cancer treatment. Here are some questions you want to make sure the patient asks:

- What is the treatment today? Do you have any fact sheets about it that I can read later?
- What are the side effects, how long do they last, what do we do to limit them?
- How are my vital signs and blood tests?
- What is the overall schedule of treatment—how often over how many months?
- Are my symptoms normal, and what can be done about them?
- What are the limits on any activity, such as driving or exercising?
- Is it okay to take _____ (vitamins, herbal supplements, aspirin, etc.)?

During this appointment, encourage your friend to be open. Leave the room if you get any sense that she wants privacy. If she seems nervous about answering the doctor's questions, for example, that might be your cue to step outside for a minute. Stand up and say "Excuse me for a moment." You don't need to say, "I think you need privacy," because that's just going to start a discussion about it. She will feel she has to urge you to stay. Just leave and stay around that door.

Survival Kits

Whenever you are keeping a patient company—to see the doctor, to have a test or a treatment—bring a bag for yourself. Keep something to drink, something to read or do, and something to eat. Drink, read, do, eat. Think about your needs for a period of several hours, or even a full day, and make sure you can be comfortable. If you happen upon one of those days when everybody in Oncology is running behind, you'll be much better company if you bring your kit. It's just like packing a diaper bag for grown-ups.

Encourage your friend to bring the same, or pack one for her. In the bag there should always be a list of medications she takes, including vitamins, over-the-counter pills, and herbal supplements. The patient should keep this list handy and up-to-date. Include the dose next to each medicine and the name and phone number of the doctor who prescribed it, plus the phone number and address of the pharmacy.

In some areas of a hospital, there will be signs asking you not to eat or drink. This is usually because other people are fasting, or because the staff doesn't want to clean up after you. Go out to the hallway if you really need to eat or drink. There will also be signs about cell phone use. Same rule applies.

Be the Chemo Buddy

Most patients need a buddy during treatments. You won't know until the first chemo treatment just what kind of buddy the patient needs. I thought my husband would be great. Five minutes later, I knew he wouldn't be. He was too worried and he looked it. I asked him to skip my treatments, and instead I asked the funniest people I know to be with me.

Chemo sessions can be short or they can take most of the day. In most cases, the patient is sitting in a recliner with a series of IV bags. Some contain chemo, some contain drugs to offset the side effects of the chemo. Today, powerful antinausea medicines have changed chemotherapy so that, again, it's not the horror that you see in movies. It's not recreational, exactly, but the medicines really help. So if you feel that your friend is trying to tough it out for some reason, tell her to quit that. Try saying something like: "The more you're relieved of side effects, the stronger you will feel and the better you will tolerate treatment, which will keep you on the recommended treatment schedule. You start letting yourself get all sick and it's going to be much harder than it needs to be."

Here's an odd thing about chemo and nausea. I can honestly tell you that chemotherapy itself never made me barf, not once. The idea of chemo, though, did, and it can still spin my stomach. It's called "anticipatory nausea," and it's a common thing. For some people, it lasts for years; every time they go back for a checkup, they feel nausea again. They feel fine otherwise, but returning to the doctor's office triggers this odd response.

I can't even listen to people talk about chemo in any detail without feeling that familiar seasickness.

You need to know the scope of the chemo treatment before you take on being a chemo buddy. If you can't sit around while somebody sits in a recliner and nods off, you will not enjoy this experience. Do another job, and leave this one to someone who likes to sit and read and chat and will bring chocolate. Remember that no cancer patient needs a vigil while they're asleep. You'll need to take breaks. Go for a walk. Get fresh air.

What Happens in Chemotherapy?

First there will be blood tests to make sure that your friend is in good shape for the treatment. These blood counts are not "normal" during chemotherapy treatment, but if they are too far from normal, treatment may have to be postponed until they are better. For example, your friend might be anemic, or showing too little ability to fight infection. This can be very difficult for the patient to deal with. She has girded herself for treatment and now has to go home and wait, possibly for another week. It's just like false labor—for both of you. The expectant mom and the husband were both geared up for this, only to be sent away. You might handle this by asking what else you can do with the patient that she might want to get done: Lunch? Errands? Movies? Shopping? Driving range?

Most of the time, everything will be fine and your friend is ready for chemo. The doses will be processed by the pharmacy in-house, generally, and this will take some time. It's not a system that you want to rush.

Chemo is usually given intravenously but may sometimes be an injection or a pill. Most patients receive the IV in the arm. Some patients have an access device implanted, kind of like a plug under the skin. Instead of having a new hole in your vein each time, they just hook you up to your plug. It is called a portocath and is usually placed in the chest. In chemotherapy, your veins sometimes get less and less cooperative as treatment goes on. The portocath is a very convenient solution. I call it my "Me Tube."

To have one installed, your friend will usually receive deep sedation and lots of local anesthetic. If he has not experienced this before, it's interesting. It's not general anesthetic and the recovery from it is much easier. He won't feel the surgery and won't remember much either. They slip a tube into a vein and a cap on the tube, all under the skin. It looks like there's a quarter under the skin and otherwise does not show. It feels a little pinchy for a week or so and after that is generally painless and you forget about it.

Because your friend will be sedated, he is going to need a ride home. The hospital will not release him to a taxi, typically. He will probably feel a little groggy and very hungry, because even for this kind of anesthesia they want the patient to fast from the night before.

Back to chemo. There will usually be a hydration bag going to keep your friend's system nice and dewy. There will be other drugs dripping in, such as antihistamines, and then the actual chemotherapy. You may be there for an hour or all day; be sure to find that out in advance so you can be prepared. You won't be helping your friend if you are anxious about the school pickup time.

In 1994, a prominent health writer, Betsy Lehman, died from a chemo overdose. Ms. Lehman wrote for the *Boston Globe* and was a highly aware and educated patient, who nonetheless was mortally harmed by error. So now, two nurses will come over with every drug your friend receives. They double-check it and triple-check it and ask the patient's name and birthday and double- and triple-check that. Don't answer the identity questions for your friend. Many of these protocols were put in place because of Betsy Lehman's death. They're essential.

Over the hours of a treatment, it's common for the patient to doze off. Some of the medicines are sedatives.

Like I said, you don't have to sit there in faithful atten-dance, but do be sure to tell your friend that you're going for a walk so that she knows where you are if she should wake up while you're out.

Many chemo chairs have a TV attached. At first, the patient thinks this is going to be great. I don't know why, but it's not. When I was in treatment, I swear that the only thing on television was a game show that gets under my skin a little and a training video called "Breastfeeding and You." You'll notice that people tend to turn the TVs up too loud because hospitals are noisy places, which is guaran-teed to irritate the people behind the neighboring curtain. So I've noticed that the TVs get less and less use as the treatment weeks go by.

People often ask me how they should behave. Just behave normally, as if you're having coffee together, except that one of you has a much more comfortable chair to recline in.

You'll notice that chemo treatment areas are friendly and informal. The procedures are strict, but the nurses and volunteers are usually very nice. You and the patient can usually get up and walk around (carefully) with the IV in tow; go to the bathroom; look out the windows.

Some patients really like to talk with other patients; some don't. You'll know quickly which way your friend likes it. It's exactly like being on a plane. You're a talker or you're not.

The side effects of chemotherapy typically do not start during this session, so you won't be seeing anything very dramatic or exciting. Your friend may just feel kind of out of it at the end.

Errands

Errands are a very intimate thing to do for someone. If I ask you to pick up my dry cleaning, you'll see what size I am, and I like to think that I've been fooling everybody. My overdue library books? You'll see what I read. My grocery list? Grocery lists are as individual as fingerprints—anybody else's looks like an alien wrote it. Canned beets? Creamed corn? You may be doing me a favor by doing the groceries, but, oh my, you'll never view me the same way again.

Helpful as it may be, however, it's generally a good idea to be very careful with anything that involves money. If mistakes can be made, they will be. If you're doing an errand that requires money, work out in advance how you're going to handle it. You might want to keep an envelope of receipts and then get a check for what you spent. You might tell your friend that you need his cash to use, or his debit card. Be clear about anything and everything that involves money, or this'll surely be when you learn that money is the quickest way to destroy a relationship.

Driving

During chemo or outpatient surgery, the patient needs drivers because there may be sedation involved. No amount of cancer is going to get her off with a judge if she hurts somebody while driving in an altered state. Doesn't matter how she got that way.

If nobody can help, check the resources in Appendix A and ask at the hospital, as there are many volunteers who drive cancer patients.

A note about carpooling errands: Carpooling might be a good errand that a cancer patient can do herself to stay connected when she's not in the midst of treatment. It can be especially good for kids if mom is still driving to soccer sometimes. Ask before you just take her off the list of volunteers.

Exercise Buddy

Very active and fit people often continue exercising during treatment. Most mortals need to reduce the intensity or frequency. Be careful if you're the exercise buddy. If you have been running together for years, you may have to slow down. Let the patient set the pace.

Be generous with your workout friend. If he has to skip workouts for now, still visit him without exercising. If you're frequent walkers, for example, give the patient the choice of walking or talking. If you just can't sit still and want every minute of your friend's social life with you to be spent walking, find another way to help the patient.

Wig Shopping

Chances are that your friend is going to lose hair. Not every kind of chemo causes hair loss, but many do.

How to handle this is highly individual. Some people try hard to hang on to every last hair, even using a technique of wrapping cold things around your head. Some people shave their heads at the first sign of hair loss. That's what I did, for two reasons. First, I hated the itchy feeling my scalp had when the hair was still there but almost falling out, and shaving relieved that. Second, I didn't want to spend any time sweeping up hair from the bed or floors or shower drain. You can help this friend by going with her for a head shaving. Usually, her regular stylist will do it for her and has possibly done it before. The stylist may recommend just going to a very short hair cut; I preferred a close shave from an electric razor. If you are doing it yourself for your friend, stick to the electric razor and don't be tempted to use a manual one, especially if you have never shaved a head before. Your experience with your legs does not count!

Many people prefer to go bald slowly. It's a more gradual adjustment. Whatever your friend decides, women usually choose to cover their heads in some way. Hats and scarves are common. You can even buy a baseball cap that has a ponytail sticking out the back.

Many women buy a wig. There are several approaches to doing this. Ask your friend's nurse if the hospital has free ones that people have donated. You can help your friend to pick her favorite, then take her to a hairdresser to have it styled. Check the Web sites in Appendix A for free wig sources. It may or may not bother your friend that someone else has worn it, but she can always wash the wig first.

If she wants to buy a new wig, there are cancer patient shops in some medical centers that provide this service. She can also go to a hair-replacement-for-women professional in your area for a truly custom wig. In any case, at some point she will want to take her wig to her own stylist.

These options are listed in order of price. Remember that many health insurance policies will reimburse your friend for part of the cost, but only if she has a prescription for the wig.

If you're the wig buddy, listen carefully to your friend. She may want to look different from how she normally looks, she may want to look the same. Just because you would want to go platinum, or curly, doesn't mean that's the right choice for her.

If most of her baldness will take place during the summer, wigs and hats feel hot or itchy. Help her to feel comfortable if she opts for going around town bald by being a supportive friend.

Childcare

Nothing is worrying your friend more than her children. Nothing is frightening her more than their future. Every time that she feels too tired to do something for them, it breaks her heart. You are going to show her that her children can be protected and cared for—in partnership with her—and that is going to accomplish more for her spirit than nearly anything else you can do. Plus, kids are just darned inconvenient and your friend is going to need plenty of help.

Many parents understand that the toughest cancer diagnosis is given to a single parent with toddlers. She is already stretched thin and cancer is going to topple everything.

Use the chart system (such as *www.lotsahelpinghands .org*) to figure out what is needed and who can help. The needs will include childcare, feeding, and driving. School-age kids will probably have friends whose parents will help out. Toddlers are more difficult if everybody works and the kids are not in preschool every day, so this can require a lot of volunteers, or one professional.

Toddlers aren't the only problem. Teenagers can react pretty extremely to a parent's cancer diagnosis. Keep an eye on them, too. If your kids are friends with their kids, step up now and make sure that they're not making any big changes, like skipping school or changing friends. You can be guaranteed that a normal teenager will not always behave better just because Mom or Dad is sick.

For school-age children, your goal is to make life as normal as possible. If there is a project to be done, offer to host the work at your house. Children can feel awful if they fall behind in school, and school-age children usually need a little help. Offer some homework sessions, help to carry the big science project, or add the child to your carpool.

Sports are a big part of many kids' lives. If you have a child on the same team, try to include the patient's child in rides, practices, even registration forms. Do the same for musical instrument classes, dance, drama.

The Pet Owner

We all rush in to help with babysitting, but some people need the most help with pets. Do everything you can to keep those pets healthy, because they will help your friend recover. For an animal lover, falling asleep with a hand on a pet's back is heavenly and stress reducing. There's plenty of research about this that has led to dogs being used in nursing homes. If you're not a pet owner, you might not believe it, but try to accept that your friend feels this way even if you don't.

Organize the pet lovers in the neighborhood to help out. Start by figuring out what this pet needs. Regular feeding or once a day? Long runs, for a big and active dog, or a quick trip to the yard for an elderly lap dog? Trips to the vet because the rabies shot is due? Keeping on top of heart-worm medicine and checking for ticks? Occupying a cat that gets destructive if left alone for too long?

You may or may not be able to walk your friend's dog. For instance, I love my friend Jane, who has two gigantic dogs who are runners. They look like they stepped out of a fairy tale to carry a giant across the Arctic. Very few people can walk them, because it requires strength and cunning. In this case, you may need to bring in a pro.

For most animals, if you are not able to walk them, just drag the teenagers in. They can clock community service hours for school. If you don't know any kids, call the local middle school and high school and ask for help. Ask if you can put up signs. If your friend can afford it, just help him to find a dog walker or pet sitter and make it easier on everybody. You can find pet care people in the yellow pages or ask at your local pet store.

Taking Care of Insurance and Billing Issues

Some patients need help with the paperwork of cancer. Health insurance can be complicated and frustrating. Unless you're an expert, or plan to become one, be careful about taking on this job. Mistakes in this field can be very expensive. General advice is that once a person is diagnosed, they should never let their health insurance lapse, because they might be unable to get back in; their ability to get life insurance just plummeted; and their ability to get long-term care insurance may be harder.

Just remember one secret about health insurance companies: It can be standard practice for them to say no to paying for something when in fact they're going to pay. Your friend, or you if you've taken on this role, will have to appeal. Don't waste too much time and spirit getting enraged when you hear "no" from the insurance company. It just means "You have to appeal this decision." Save your rage for a second appeal.

If you can't help with this job, and nobody else can, your friend may need a patient advocate or social worker. Talk with the hospital to see what resources they have.

The Medicine Buddy

Managing prescriptions fits into the same category. If you're able to help, great, but only help if you're really able to.

One task is to fill a daily or weekly medicine box. This is a risky job but can be a very important one. First, insist that the doctor give your friend a printout of medications, with the doses and schedule. A handwritten list is not enough; a list dictated over the phone isn't either. After every appointment, ask for a new and dated printout. Do not fill the medicine boxes by following the pharmacy labels; follow the doctor's schedule. Tell the doctor and pharmacy about any differences between the two.

If you take on the job of helping with medicines, be sure that your friend is capable of taking them on the right schedule. It doesn't help for you to fill up the cute little plastic boxes only to have her take them all at once. With some forms of chemotherapy, the pills you take before you get there are very important. If your friend is not capable of doing that, please talk with the doctor about it. It may be time for visiting nurses. Or for a family member to take charge.

Remember that a good pharmacist is a treasure to keep. They will help you bypass paperwork when you need a two-week supply for your friend to go on vacation; they will help with any conflicts between medicines; they can be a wonderful resource. Most of the time, pharmacists will allow you to pick up prescriptions for your friend, but be sure to bring your driver's license for identification. You may need a letter of permission from your friend for some medicines, such as pain relievers.

A few times during treatment, I had to have medicines blended up. This means that they don't come in pill or liquid form ready-made for the pharmacist. There's mouth rinse for sores, for example, that is a combination of several ingredients. The pharmacy did not carry it and does not mix, or "compound," medicines. You can help your friend by finding the pharmacy in your area that "compounds." Most pharmacies don't. Your doctor may know which pharmacy still compounds medicines, but the pharmacist is probably the best source. It's a good thing to know. You know who else might know who compounds? The veterinarian!

Pain Relief Management

Plenty of people—especially older women, in my experience—think they don't want any pain medication. If your friend resists pain medication, ask the staff to talk with her about it and answer her questions. If you have to, tell her how aggravating she is while in pain. Maybe that'll get her to get some relief. You can guarantee that she's harboring fears about pain relief if she won't take any.

Some people have heard horror stories about constipation. Many people can handle cancer like it's a cold, but live in dread of constipation. I don't know why, but doctors often forget to tell patients about the importance of taking softeners while on certain medications.

Whatever you do, remember that all pain medication should be kept in a locked box at home. You can get one for your friend from an office supply store. There are plenty of people who take pain medication to get high, not to relieve pain, and that's a good way to develop a big problem. These folks are not above stealing from cancer patients. Lock the stuff up. Tell your friend to hide the key. No, you can't always trust the resident teenagers or their friends.

Some people who don't want pain medication are actually afraid of addiction, since many pain medications have narcotics in them. It used to be that everyone worried about patients becoming addicted, and some doctors just didn't want to prescribe any narcotics. Thankfully, that view has changed. These days, the typical doctor believes that if you are prone to addiction you will have developed signs of that before now; that pain medication taken when in pain is unlikely to cause addiction or even a narcotic "high"; and that the body can heal itself better when not racked with pain. So for most people, addiction is not an issue.

Be sure your friend takes a stool softener, though. That side effect is real.

Patient Advocacy

What is the patient advocate's job? It can be a thousand different things, depending on your friend's condition and personality, your personality, the hospital, the doctor, the nurses, the food service workers.

Let's start with how hospitals would view you as a "patient advocate." At its most basic level, patient advocacy means observing the patient's needs and making sure they are met. Patient advocacy can mean making sure that everything done for your friend is done correctly. It can mean pestering nurses and doctors. Perhaps the patient's pain level has spiked and he needs a new plan for pain management. Maybe he is just cold and needs a blanket. It can mean that you will be asking for things for the patient, pushing for things, demanding things. How much your friend needs this depends on what shape he is in and what his personality is. You can read more about this in the "Doctor Buddy" section. Many people who don't like conflict are very uncomfortable with the patient advocate job and should not volunteer to take it on. It can mean being persistent with doctors and nurses and not everyone likes that. Advocacy can also mean helping out if the patient has an uncooperative insurance plan, or none at all. It can mean badgering them every step of the way. Unless you are an expert in this field, though, see if the hospital has a professional to help you figure out this minefield.

Advocacy can also mean researching sources to help pay for medical bills. Even if your friend has health insurance, there are going to be co-pays or deductibles that can add up quickly. Appendix B offers some sites that can coach you on how to help under these circumstances.

As a last resort, you might also be the friend who organizes a fundraiser for the patient's family. He may have a lifetime limit, for example, of a million dollars that his insurance will cover. Your community, school, or house of worship may want to chip in by hosting a potluck dinner, for example, or a road race.

Advocacy can take many other forms. In a political sense it inspires many friends of cancer patients. You may find yourself writing letters to Congress about mandatory hospital stays for cancer surgery, or family leave bills. Your friend will feel appreciative, but will not always join you. Some patients are stirred and inspired to lead a lifetime of cancer fundraising and advocacy. Others leave the last day of treatment and never want to hear about cancer again. It's your friend's choice, and yours too.

What You Can Teach Your Friend about Help

Cancer patients usually need this simple but profound wake-up call: "Your loved ones need to help you because it will make them feel better. It is an act of generosity and love to let them be helpful." Most cancer patients need that reminder just about every day.

So when a neighbor calls and offers to trim the hedges, encourage your friend to say *yes*. No more guilt-ridden self-reliance. She needs help, and her friends and loved ones *need* to help. This is a glorious time when everyone's needs match. Besides, she'll have her turn, someday, to help everyone who helps her now.

If she has trouble understanding how it is really an act of kindness to accept help, ask her about times in her past that she has wanted to help another person. Most people will have a sudden flash of recognition.

If your friend is still trying to go it alone, you can always try the guilt alarm: Remind her of the burden on her spouse and kids, or on her parents. She might not be noticing that everyone is pitching in and she might not know that they all could use a break. So when a neighbor comes by with a lawn mower and her spouse looks relieved, tell her not to turn the neighbor away.

CARE ALERT

You may be tempted to deliver your meal on your fanciest china, with linen napkins, a tablecloth, and a vase of flowers. Remember: Nobody, not even you, should use containers that have to be returned!

Chapter Eight

The Toolbox of Soulful Ways to Help

By NOW, A team is in place to care for your friend's physical well-being. How about the rest of her? In this toolbox, you're bringing out all of the ways in which you can help her strengthen her spirit.

Company

Keeping a friend company is a wonderful gift you can give, but I promise it will take some time to figure out what is best. You'll know a lot more after your first visit. If you're exhausting the friend, you need to refine what you're doing. One friend wants you to talk, or sing, another friend needs a quiet companion or prayer. Some people like a hand held, a foot rubbed, hair brushed; other people can't stand any of that.

How do you find out which kind of friend you have? Go along, keep her company, and then ask. If you don't know this friend well enough to ask, you don't belong there keeping her company.

Try saying this: "I want to be good company for you, so I'm going to ask you if you like something or not, and I need you to tell me so I don't drive you crazy. I mean that. I need you to be honest with me."

It's a good idea to know yourself really well before you visit someone who's really not feeling well. Do you have trouble sitting still? Do you have to fold laundry or check your e-mail or make phone calls anytime you sit in a chair? Then choose your type of visit carefully. Your friend knows you and may dread spending an hour with you, if she thinks you are going to run around the house straightening pictures, washing dishes, and sorting the mail. Talk honestly with her to figure out how you can be most helpful.

Be a Good Ear

Most patients need to talk about their experiences and their feelings. A group of friends can take turns being the listener, but step up if you're particularly good at this.

A good listener is paying attention, not daydreaming. A good listener is not judging, but is taking it all in and is feeling empathetic or sympathetic. You can fake being a good listener, but not for long. Being a good listener requires you to be a loving, caring person who is able to put yourself aside and really hear someone. If you just pretend to be, you will be found out eventually.

But the cancer patient has to understand that his friends are not therapists, and a group of friends is not a support group. Life is going on for the group of friends, and the cancer patient should understand that. He will probably not want to hear anybody whining, but encourage him to try to listen to his friends as he normally would.

The same good ideas apply to how you listen to a friend with cancer as how you listen to a friend who is grieving or celebrating. It's his feelings that matter right now, not your opinions. If the roles were reversed, you would be entitled to the same treatment. So try to listen without judging.

Be Careful about Giving Advice and Guidance If You've Had Cancer Before

Ah, you think, how great it will be for your friend, that you've had cancer too. It can be. Maybe you're a good example of the end of treatment, the return to normal life. Maybe you kept yourself from hysteria most of the time, or had a terrific attitude, or finished chemo without missing a day of work. Maybe you're just a simply great person who happens to have had cancer, who knows a lot about it. That can be great for your friend and she will seek you out.

But it can also be exactly like seeing your neighbor, a mother of one baby, when you're pregnant. She might be lovely and joyful, she might be informative and supportive, or she might be a know-it-all who makes you wonder what you're going to turn into after your own baby is born. Because she's gone ahead of you, it's going to be that way forever. She is going to have the perfect toddler, the perfect kindergartener, school-ager—you get the idea.

Same thing with cancer. Think carefully about your listening skills before you even talk with your newly diagnosed friend. You will be sorely tempted to think you know everything she's feeling and to tell her that. Resist the temptation—she still has to get through this herself.

Be extremely careful about medical advice. Your cancer is not the same as hers, even if it seems exactly alike. You aren't clones, even if you're twins.

No matter how certain you are that the patient should follow the same course you did, count to a million before you speak. You can't know what's right for him, except this: Urge him to get a second opinion. Offer to go with him. But don't think that having had cancer makes you an oncologist. It's dangerous for him and for your friendship.

My advice: Use your experience to help him to identify what might be issues. Would he opt for a lower chance of recurrence or a higher risk of side effects? If the treatment runs the risk of impotence or incontinence, how bad would that be for him? Suggest listing the positives and negatives and taking time to think about them.

I can only tell people what I did and what I think the issues are. They're truly different for everybody, and you don't know for sure until you've done it. Think for a moment if you've had a mastectomy, for example. Let's say you now develop cancer in your other breast. Would you make the same decisions now that you did for your first cancer? Maybe, maybe not. I don't think you can be that certain. So you certainly can't offer certainty to your friend.

So listen as much as possible, ask as much as possible. Keep reminding her that you can only explain what you did and why, you can't make the decision for her. Treatment and reconstruction decisions are entirely personal and nobody can make them for another.

Prayer

I like to call myself a God-fearing atheist, but cancer taught me something about the power of prayer. When particular people were praying for me, I could tell. I could feel it. I felt a real sense of being carried through treatment by prayer.

People sent Mass cards, signed me up in prayer groups, came over and prayed with me. I loved having people pray who were of different religions—just in case, because you never know.

Most people want your prayers. Some people don't. I don't really know why. If somebody tells you he really doesn't like "the whole prayer thing," keep praying, but do it privately. Some patients and friends like to pray together just before starting treatment or having surgery. In my opinion, doctors and nurses should accommodate prayer and they usually do. Out of courtesy, you should keep your prayer brief. You should not try to hold hands if everybody has already scrubbed up. Also, it's polite to keep your prayer nice. Don't ask the whole operating room for a moment of silence so you can say a loud prayer for God to open the heart of your godless, unbaptized, unconfirmed, uncircumcised surgeon.

If your friend is staying in the hospital, and he believes in the power of prayer, be sure he checks off the religion box on the admitting forms. I once checked off all of the boxes and had visits from three major religions. You never know. Maybe you and your friend are of different faiths and you worry about causing a problem by expressing yours. Let me have a minute on the soapbox here: It is good for all of us to witness and share in how we all worship. If your friend doesn't feel that way, he probably can't be taught right now. But if you are both open to faith-sharing even if you sing from different hymn books, you'll find this a deeply enriching spiritual journey together.

How to start? Ask your friend what his favorite prayer is, or his favorite scripture passage. Most religions have prayers, scripture, meditations, or readings. You cannot offend anybody by asking this. Listen carefully, ask for a translation if necessary. Then share yours.

If you feel a strong need to read from the Bible, you can always stick to the Psalms. They are universally loved and awfully inspiring and comforting at the same time.

Plan a Trip Together

Many people with cancer want to travel as soon as they feel better. My oncologist at Beth Israel Deaconess Medical Center, Lowell Schnipper, says some people benefit from planning a trip while in treatment and then taking it when feeling well again.

If you're good traveling friends together, planning a trip would be fun. Buy trip insurance in case you have to cancel. I'm not saying that to be pessimistic, you just never know. Some people bounce back quickly at the end of radiation, some take awhile. While the idea of traveling together might be just what your friend needs, there are many precautions to take and issues to consider when you are planning your trip.

Being a Travel Buddy during treatment is different from touring Costa Rica six months after radiation is finished. You can be sure that nobody in chemotherapy likes to be too far from indoor plumbing. Your friend who loves wilderness camping might want a roof and a bathroom this time. Diarrhea is a common side effect and you don't have to have cancer to know that your anxiety level hits the moon if you're out and about while so afflicted.

She will need to stay hydrated, so make sure you make plenty of stops even if she doesn't think she needs it. She may need to be taking medication on a schedule, with food or water, or on an empty stomach, so be sure that you think about that before heading too far from civilization.

People with sensitive stomachs feel better with smaller meals. If your friend has some breakthrough nausea despite all of the medications to prevent it, be sure to try the small meal strategy. It's also a good idea to think bland. Because chemotherapy attacks the cells that multiply the fastest, and there are plenty of those along the way your food travels, the digestive system can take a beating. Sometimes she will feel as if she's sore all the way through her system. Good thing you don't have pain nerves in the colon, isn't it? But her mouth and the route to her stomach may be a little raw. Not everyone has that experience, so if your friend feels that she can handle whatever she wants to eat, don't hover or nag. Just be watchful.

Remember that anyone in chemotherapy should carry a medical sheet. It should have the phone numbers of the doctors and a list of medications and doses. It should list what kind of chemotherapy is being taken. It should say what to do in an emergency. It's not that I can think of any particular chemo-related emergencies, I just think when you're receiving a challenging treatment you can save yourself a lot of time if you have your information with you. Your friend might even want to carry a letter authorizing you to make medical decisions. It should be dated for the time period you're traveling together.

> **" I loved it when my friend . . . "**
>
> ". . . Saved coupons for me from my favorite stores that I would have missed otherwise."
>
> ". . . Washed the dirty window near my favorite chair so I would have sunlight and a view."
>
> ". . . Gave me a box of quarters because the only parking at my house is metered. It made me feel better when people were doing me favors that at least I could ask my kids to run out and fill the meter."

And, while you're traveling, you're allowed to remind all and sundry of the rank God has assigned for seats on buses and trains. Frail, handicapped and elderly people are first, followed closely by pregnant women. Pregnant women who are getting toward those last days trump nearly everybody else. People with temporary injuries as shown by a cast are next. Cancer patients are right behind them. Children, contrary to popular opinion, come last.

Being in a Crowd

Many chemotherapy patients have little resistance to germs. Chemo compromises the immune system and can make it easy to catch other people's bugs. Your friend may have to avoid a lot of contact, including air travel. Some patients even avoid kisses and hugs.

Carry some hand sanitizer with you just in case. If you are traveling to visit other people, be sure to find out if anyone there is sick or contagious. Be careful around children, because they travel in germ-ridden packs of wild mammals. Help your friend to avoid as many germs as possible if her resistance is low. You definitely do not want her to be out of town and sick.

Hot Flashes and Chills

Some chemotherapy can cause brand-new hormonal side effects. She may be young folk, but she can still get the symptoms of menopause during treatment. Bring layers of clothing along on your trip together, because your friend may be sweating one moment and freezing the next. She (or he) will be turning on the air conditioning in the car in

North Dakota in January and won't even wonder if you're chilly. Bring layers.

Hormonal side effects are famous among women, but men get them too from certain treatments. Scientists know that the coldest place on earth is a bedroom containing two hormonally disadvantaged people of either gender.

Men, however, get made fun of for it. It's supposed to be a girl thing. So don't be surprised if your male friend is suffering in silence. That is something men know how to do. Women, not so much, but we're a lot funnier about it.

Music

If you want to give a really big gift to a cancer patient, make it an MP3 player with comfortable headphones. Put music and audio books on it and invite friends and family to send their own contributions. Cancer patients spend a lot of time sitting still during treatment and testing. An MP3 player gives them a world to retreat into. Walk around the chemo area and see the number of very relaxed looking people who have the telltale white wires.

If an MP3 player is too much money, get a cheap CD player. Give the patients CDs, and don't expect to get them back. If this is a popular idea with the patient, you can let everybody know to send CDs instead of other gifts.

An MP3 player is also a great project for the office to do together for a colleague; everyone can chip in to buy a small one and fill it with favorite songs.

Giving music is a little bit like giving books; you'll never know if what you like is what they will like. Your jazz might be fingernails on a blackboard to your friend. Don't worry—this is a time when it really is the thought that counts. Your friend's taste may surprise you. Some people find that they don't want to associate their favorite things with cancer treatment. I'm one of those; for my first treatment I brought one of my favorite books, then realized I would be reminded of chemotherapy every time I picked it up in the future. I never brought it again. So, your friend might be even more inclined to try some new music at this point in her life.

Noise-reducing headphones make a great music-related gift for a cancer patient too. You can also just lend a pair if you own them. Hospitals are noisy and noise is tiring, especially at night. Those headphones can be a peaceful oasis.

Be the Communicator

It used to be that nobody would know your friend had cancer. People didn't want to say the word. It's different now. In most countries, people are open about having cancer.

But communicating about it isn't always easy. Let's start by saying that "communications" means "staying in touch with important people without getting worn out."

When you had a baby during the dark ages, it took at least three days to call everybody you had to call. Weeks later, you sent an announcement with a little photo to everyone you hadn't called.

Today, you have an e-mail distribution list ready. You have a digital camera. The baby's picture is up on the hospital Web site before he has even peed. You still call a few people, but far fewer than you had to a generation ago.

Your friend might communicate about cancer via e-mail. It's a very good way to let everybody know what's happening. It lets people feel connected, without exhausting the patient with phone calls. Some patients prefer to have a central place for information, such as *www.carepages.com* or *www.caringbridge.org*. Others worry too much about privacy to do that. Let the patient decide and remember that there will always be friends and relatives who are not Web-savvy.

Some patients head in the opposite direction and want nobody knowing anything. If they're simply private, fine. Sometimes, though, they would welcome an offer to handle communication for them. If you can help out by keeping people informed for them, be sure to. Just be careful about family dynamics under these circumstances. If your friend just wants you to keep his alarmist and hypochondriac aunt from talking to him, you need to know that from the beginning.

Answering the phone in a cancer patient's home can be a full-time and exhausting task. Everyone wants to hear the same story about the surgery, for example, and ask the same questions. There are three gifts you can give to a patient who doesn't have these: caller ID service from the phone company, a cordless phone that will show caller ID in the handset and on the base, and an answering machine. These will help you or the patient to answer the calls you need to answer and skip the ones you don't, or to call someone back when it's most convenient.

Do yourself a favor and be very careful how widely you give out anybody's cell phone number.

Blogging

Writing can be very therapeutic. Your friend might love to have a journal to keep, or may send volumes of e-mails. It provides a place to unload or process feelings, and it is useful for tracking change and progress. While a beautiful volume is still the favorite tool for many people, more and more cancer patients are blogging. If you have volunteered to set up a blog for your friend, there are plenty of instructions online, none of which I have ever figured out, but apparently it's easy to do. My highly technical method is to ask the teenager in the family to do it. Try *www.blogger.com*, *www.carepages.com*, or *www.caringbridge.org* for a free and easy way to start.

If blogging is new to your friend, be sure to remind her of a few warnings. Blogs are public and permanent. If you don't want your boss, any future boss, or your neighbors following the details of your illness, you don't keep a blog.

Don't say anything on your blog that would identify you to strangers. This sounds obvious but many, many people make this mistake. Having said all of that, a patient blog is where you can freely spout or carefully edit your thoughts, feelings, and experiences. This can be a wonderful outlet. Let everyone know your friend's Web address and invite them to comment.

If your friend is keeping a blog, she will love it when people leave comments. For most bloggers though, no matter how many friends and family you have, you don't get a lot of response. There are people who spend little time online and would rather call. Help your friend to understand that a silent blog is a very common thing. Many, many patients write the blog just for themselves and any comments are nice unexpected surprises.

One patient I know sends out an e-mail to his family and friends anytime he adds something to the blog. This will encourage people to visit it, but your friend may still be disappointed if not everybody does. Remind him that he's doing the writing for *him*.

Encourage your friend to keep writing no matter what. People will say it's therapeutic, and it is. For me it was a way to organize my approach to cancer. It helped me to get my mind around what my way was going to be.

Keep in Touch from Afar

It's awful living far away from a close friend or relative with cancer. You're going to miss each other terribly now. This is a very good time to take advantage of answering machines and e-mail. Leave her a message, a brief one, to tell her hello and that you're thinking of her. E-mail her a quick thought almost daily. Send her a noncancer joke if you can't think of anything to say. Don't worry if you don't hear back all the time. Communicating can be overwhelming and you may have to settle for the group e-mails.

If you have a boatload of inspiration e-mails you have received, please don't just "forward" them. You know what I mean. You receive an e-mail that has been forwarded forty-seven times. You scroll through pages of names, you get to the bottom and it just says "Smile." So instead of forwarding, copy and paste the actual message into a clean, fresh new e-mail.

Don't forget regular mail. Send a note, a card, some photos. People often ask me what kind of card they should send if a person is terminally ill. You don't send the one with the balloon on it saying "Just 'popped' by to say get well soon!" You send a beautiful picture card and you write in it that you're thinking of her and sending much love. Or use stationery and skip the card.

If you want to schedule a trip to visit with your out-of-town friend, talk with her about timing. You may be aching to take care of her during treatment. She may be aching for something different, maybe to have a fun escape at the end of treatment. Talk together to see if you can do what you both want to do. If you can't, she gets to pick this time.

If you do go to visit, is it more helpful for you to stay with her or at a hotel? Can you help with chores at home, or at least keep from making more of them? Are you prepared to have to share your visit with other friends and family? Do you get along really well with her spouse or should you keep your distance if you can't make it work?

Staying with anybody requires open and honest communication. She may be very uncomfortable about sharing a bathroom right now, for example, if she's recovering from surgery and has to do a lot of preparation in order to take a shower. She may not want the washing machine going constantly, even if you're helping by doing laundry. She may not want the smell of cooking, even if you have offered to make a month of frozen meals. Be open to her thoughts and ask how things are going as time goes by.

Distraction

Everybody needs a break from his or her problems. Here's the catch: If you tell me "I'm going to take you swimming so we can get your mind off of cancer," guess what will happen? I will think of nothing but cancer. I will float around asking you if you think salt water, or chlorine, or bathing caps, or flip flops, or sunscreen might be carcinogenic.

Instead, first think of something distracting to do with your friend. Suggest the plan, without referring to cancer at all. He will be suspicious and will ask you if you're trying to get his mind off cancer. "No," you can say honestly. "I'm trying to get *my* mind off of cancer."

You can probably think of specific activities that your friend would enjoy without any help, but here are some of the most distracting things to do:

- A funny movie. A happy musical.
- A play that is so depressing it makes you realize how lucky you all really are. Seriously. Sit down for a little dramatic contemporary theater and you will find out that you're both the picture of mental health.

- Lunch, if food is appealing.
- Shopping.
- Golf, with a cart.
- Visit an old mutual friend (especially one neither of you particularly likes who is in poor health and makes you feel like thanking your lucky stars!).
- A new sport that is thrilling. Parasailing, for example, or maybe croquet, it doesn't matter.
- Doing something for someone who needs help. No better distraction than that.

Keep a Positive Attitude
(and Nudge Your Friend Toward One)

People love to talk about this around cancer patients. By week three after diagnosis, your friend is going to snap and scream, "I would feel much more positive if every negative person I know wasn't lecturing me to have a positive attitude!"

I do believe in the power of attitude. I believe in it not because it cures cancer, because it doesn't. I just think it helps patients to keep going back for treatment and to reduce stress. Those are major good reasons.

Every once in a while somebody in the medical field likes to do a study about positive attitudes, proving they're not important, or they are important. I wish they'd quit that. The truth is, I've seen positive people die from cancer, and I've seen negative people live forever. You can find a study to prove anything you want.

Instead, ask an oncologist if having a positive attitude is important. They'll say yes. They've all seen it—the person who can will him- or herself to endure very difficult treatment. It's hard for a doctor to say that something is true if it can't be proven scientifically. Still, oncologists often see the power of sheer optimism.

But what is a positive attitude? It takes a different form in everybody. With some, it's serene and even meditative. For others it's physical vitality. Or a broad smile and a confident walk. I think a positive attitude is simply this: loving life, wanting to keep living it; doing whatever it takes to keep living a healthy life; not spending time complaining and despairing; being a role model for others.

Still, your friend could walk around in a dress made out of smiley buttons and somebody is still going to lecture her to have a positive attitude. As with all irritating things that are going to happen during treatment and in everyday life forever, she has a choice.

First, she can try to think of people who say thoughtless things as handing her a little bit of string. What happens next? Well, she can wind her strings of irritation into a great big ball of irritation and carry it around with her, burdening her with a heavy weight. Or she can hand it back to each person who contributes to it. Encourage her to say something along the lines of: "I've got that covered, thanks." I don't know why this helps, but it does.

If you feel that your friend really is letting her negative thoughts drag her down, how can you shake her out of it? You can't. She's acting like a teenager and she needs time to grow out of it.

You can be a good role model of positive thinking yourself and lead the conversation to good news in her life; when she is ready, ask her if she is ready to come to the surface for air.

Tell her you know she has been despairing for lots of good reasons and tell her you're worried that despair will hurt her, that it will leave her depressed. Tell her you think she's ready to come up from the depths and get a good lungful of air and a bath of sunlight.

When you do something with love and with respect, it is usually not a lecture and it will often be well received.

> **" I loved it when my friend . . . "**
>
> ". . . Gave me a great big tray with sides so I could have drinks and food in bed and not fuss if it spilled. I think it was some kind of 'flying saucer'–type sled!"
>
> ". . . Helped my spouse learn to make a fresh clean bed for when I came home from the hospital."
>
> ". . . Photographed every stage of the treatment. My friend is a great photographer."
>
> ". . . Did not take a single photograph during any stage of the treatment even though she is a great photographer."

Offer a Moment of Normalcy

A normal day doesn't sound like a big gift, but it is. It is a positive reminder that life goes on, with you or without you, and it may as well be with you. I have a favorite example. My friend Laura and I both lost our mothers to melanoma. Marian, Laura's mom, was told on a Monday that hers had reached her brain. That night, while Marian's kids were frantically looking for her to console her, to cry with her, to comfort her and each other, she wasn't home. She had gone bowling. "Monday is my bowling night," she said. Our mothers both taught us some important lessons about how to die, and this was a big one.

So we went bowling after my first chemo treatment in honor of Marian. I thought Laura should let me win, now that I had cancer for pity's sake. But she didn't. This was a gift, a major gift: a day of normal life. Laura beats me at everything, except I can eat more in a sitting. That day of bowling symbolizes what I treasure from Laura, that she made life go on for me and made me feel as normal as possible, whether I wanted to or not.

Give the same gift to your friend. Do something you've always done together and treat him as you always have. Don't let him win.

As with everything, be sure your plans are a good fit with the treatment schedule. Maybe you normally go to the movies, but the doctor wants your friend to avoid crowds because his immune system is compromised. So you go to an uncrowded matinee and bring hand sanitizer, or rent a video and make popcorn.

Make Her Laugh

Cancer is not at all funny, but life continues to be so even under stress. The idea of laughing about life with cancer is something only cancer patients can deeply appreciate. Everyone else gets nervous. They're so often anxious about offending a patient, when in fact the patient is desperate for levity.

Laughter stimulates the endocrine system and the pituitary gland, releases the body's natural painkillers, decreases muscle tension and can boost the immune system. This is not wishful thinking but an established observation by doctors and nurses, now the subject of research.

Doctors and nurses know the healing effects of laughter, but they're rarely all that funny. "You should laugh a lot," they say in a voice that sounds like a very depressed ghost, "and here's your chemo schedule."

I was very fortunate to come across funny medical people. One day my oncologist—a revered chief of oncology—arrived with a team of students. He asked if they could join us for my exam. Yes, I said, but if I have to be topless, so does everyone. My dignified doctor loosened his tie. The students paled and I laughed deeply. When my surgeon had a knife in my back, I asked him if he's ever grossed out when cutting into someone. "Oh, yes," he said, "that's why I keep my eyes closed."

I've heard over and again how tired cancer patients are of the melodrama, of the victim mentality of cancer. They like to laugh about life. Not about cancer, but about ordinary life that has cancer in it.

Try bringing a portable DVD player and a funny movie to a treatment. Give her a funny book. Yes, it's true that one person's joke may not be another's. But you know each other as friends, so you probably know what makes her laugh, and if you get it wrong, she will forgive you.

But skip the cancer jokes. Stick to life.

Gifts?

Think carefully about whether you should give a patient gifts or not. Chances are high that your friend does not need guest towels with cancer ribbons on them. In general, gifts that will be lasting reminders of an event should be reserved for happy events, like births, not for having your testicles removed.

If the patient will be hospitalized for several days, flowers that arrive on day one are cheery. Flowers received on the last day are silly. They're impossible to bring home, though they might be nice for another patient. Some patients feel that flowers are for funerals, so always find out if the patient likes flowers before you send them.

Don't bring anything that is heavy or awkward, like big books or big pictures in frames, unless you'll be taking them home for the patient yourself. My friend Jane is a gift genius: She gives you what she would normally give you if cancer were not involved. So she'll bring something funny, or delicious, or beautiful, not a big ceramic cancer ribbon.

If you live in a snowy place, taking up a collection for a plowing service is a great gift for anyone with an illness. Same for the fall cleanup of the yard, or the spring cleanup, or the summer mowing.

If someone loves books and magazines, send them. I enjoy getting magazines that I would never normally read—or at least I never admit to reading them. One of my sisters collected every rag you can buy at the checkout counter and it was a feast for me. So consider sending silly magazines. Or magazines that your friend loves but does not want to spend the money on.

Video games are frowned upon in some circles, but they can be good gifts. Yes, avoid all of the horrible, evil ones. But some games can be a good distraction. And sometimes, a kid wants to be with Dad but is uncomfortable and doesn't want to talk. Hand her a small handheld game system such as a Nintendo DS and a few games and she can sit and keep Dad company (if Dad doesn't start playing it himself!).

I've already suggested that you avoid cancer-related gifts. It's possible to spend serious money on ribbon jewelry. You can even buy ribbon earrings of gold and diamonds. There must be somebody who likes the idea, but most patients I know don't want a little cancer sign hanging off their ears. For most everybody I know, if you hand them a jewelry box, it'd better contain something they would actually wear.

" I loved it when my friend . . . "

". . . Organized group things that would make me feel like I was still connected—like everybody from the office sent a song for my iPod based on a theme, or a CD. Everybody from the office sent a favorite joke."

". . . Reminded my kids to bring in the newspaper. To load the dishwasher. To empty the dishwasher."

". . . Taught my kids how to do laundry."

Gifts are really not called for at all, but some people like to send a gift when treatment is finished. Make it personal, not about cancer. A happy card. Stationery. Chocolate. A box of golf balls. A new game. If you want to send a small gift while your friend is still in treatment, try sending a neck roll that is designed for dozing off in a chair; a warm, portable blanket such as *www.eaglecreek.com*'s comfort travel blanket, which rolls up into a pillow and has a zippered pocket in it; or a magazine subscription that is light and entertaining.

Hospital Visits

Everyone is different about how to behave when someone is in the hospital. From culture to culture, the traditions vary greatly. In some families, everyone is expected to hang out at the hospital at all hours and then bring food to the patient's house. In others, only the immediate family even knows about the hospitalization.

The hospital likes visits from friends to be kept short. This is a good idea usually but not always. Once when my father was in the hospital, the nurse on duty insisted that we only visit one at a time. She had not seen how loud we could be, she just knew that my father had eight children, and wanted to stop us right away. So even the siblings who had traveled from far away could not sit by my dad. Eventually, we ignored her. She was very controlling and very wrong at the same time, an awful combination.

Listen to the hospital's policies, but don't feel they're commandments. If your mother is near death and you just flew in from Tokyo, don't stop at the door just because the sign says that visiting hours are over. Most hospitals mean "Visiting hours are over if you're awful and noisy."

Above all, don't ask if you may bring your children. No. Don't ask any question that your friend would be too polite to decline. If she wants to see your children, she'll ask. The only people who ask to see children in a hospital are parents and sometimes grandparents. In today's medical climate, a person actually spending the night in the hospital is usually pretty sick or recovering from surgery. With some cancer treatments, however, it's a little bit different. Your friend might be hospitalized for treatments and be feeling pretty good most of the time. In that case, he'll be wanting company and distraction. Plan ahead with him and then see what works best.

Interacting with the Family

It's time to talk about how you relate to your friend's family. If you want to be a helpful contributor to your friend's soulful life, her family is key. More than ever in her life, her family's many assets and foibles will be in play and will be very close to her heart.

There is nothing about it that I can predict for you, except that everyone will be more intense than usual. The self-centered daughter who expects Mom to take care of her kids? She'll ask for money to pay for childcare. The generous one who takes care of everyone? She'll work herself to the point of illness. The greedy one? He'll be scoping out your friend's jewelry for his girlfriend.

People do surprise you when someone has cancer. Weak people might rise to the test; strong people might not do a thing. Your friend's family may be wonderful; they may be awful. If they're wonderful, you're not even reading this section. You're reading it because maybe your friend's beloved family has done an awful thing or two. It's the awful ones who are, of course, the most fun to talk about.

Talking about them is probably the only thing you will be able to do; you may not be able to change anything, no matter how much you want to. It's very painful, for example, for you to see your friend's children or siblings treat him badly. You know that if you step in, you'll be caught in the cross fire and none of these people will end up speaking to you.

That's the choice you have to make. If you're willing to take the heat, and you're convinced it's essential for your friend's happiness, comfort, or safety, go ahead and throw a few grenades. Tell those kids and siblings how to help the patient and tell them what they need to stop doing. Tell the greedy one to put everything back. Tell the self-centered one to grow up. Tell the generous one to go home, she's just helping her lazy siblings to become even lazier.

You of course can do this in the nicest possible way. You can coax, cajole, and coo. In my experience, one way or the other, these people will not like you. There is a special section of heaven for people like you if you decide to jump in. "Blessed are the troublemakers," God says, "for they will make that awful bunch of spoiled brats shut up."

How do you help the family if your friend is terminally ill? Family dynamics when someone dies are a complex thing. Since this book is about you as the patient's friend, the best advice I can give you is to stay away from the family dynamics. Their relationships are going to be more intense and their friction is going to be worse; they have only begun down a road that might bring them closer or might drive them apart. Skip it. If you decide to get involved because you think you can bring a level head to a tense process, go ahead if you believe you can help. Just plan at least two escape routes.

Helping Your Friend Manage the Long-Distance Family

Two areas need management for your friend who has a long-distance family: the phone and the houseguest. You'll read this more than once in this book: If your friend does not have a cordless phone, caller ID, an answering machine, and a ringer you can turn off, these are wonderful gifts. The phone can be a wonderful thing or a constant intrusion. There will be wonderful people calling with good wishes and some not-so-wonderful needy folks who will wear your friend out.

For special out-of-towners, the phone is a wonderful tool. When my father was in the last few days of his life, many family members called and one of us in the room would hold the phone to his ear. It wasn't that he could carry on a conversation, but he could listen. He could hear a prayer or a thank you or an I Love You. I think it was a great gift for him and for the callers.

As for the houseguest, anybody who expects to stay in a patient's house had better be extremely close or extremely competent. Otherwise, the out-of-towner must stay somewhere else. If your friend has out-of-towners who expect to stay with him, help him by being the mean one who says no. Your only concern is your friend. If he wants a house full of guests, great. If not, but he's unable to say no, I don't care if you have to wrap the bedroom doors in that yellow crime-scene tape. You can really help by telling the out-of-towners that it just has to be quiet so the decision is for nobody to stay. If you can, offer to house the out-of-towner who has nowhere else to stay.

I hope your friend is blessed with loving family and friends among the out-of-towners. If so, help them to stay in touch. Help your friend by managing e-mails, blogs, phone calls, and letters. This is a wonderful gift to give him.

CARE ALERT

Are you helping too much? Too much help is bad for everybody. Everyone who loves this patient needs to be helping. Her family needs to be helping most of all. So be careful that you don't wear yourself out—but even more important, be sure you're not weakening everybody's responsibilities by doing too much.

Chapter Nine

When Your Relationship
Presents Special Challenges

✐❤

SOME RELATIONSHIPS ARE friendships, of a kind, but have special challenges. Sometimes they create many emotional issues for you—as when a sibling has cancer. Sometimes they require you to take on a difficult role—as when an in-law you don't get along with has cancer and needs your help. Think about your child's teacher—you want to help her, but you also want her to keep doing her job well. Same goes for the school bus driver, your hair stylist, your attorney—many, many people in your life. Employees, bosses, and colleagues all also require some special thought.

When Your Sibling Has Cancer

Having a sibling with cancer is an especially awful feeling. You love this person. Your relationship might be simple or complicated, but you love them. Their sickness reminds you of your own mortality and of your childhood, good or bad. It's going to be very complicated for you to sort out your own feelings, while at the same time trying to muster your strength to help out.

If a younger sibling is sick, you will likely feel especially moved. You may feel very protective, you may feel strong needs to make her get better. If the patient is the eldest, you may feel scared. It may feel as if your family is aging, or maybe that the strongest one is weakening. These are paths your family will have to take in life, but cancer has made it happen all too soon. It can help to remind yourself that you are facing a life challenge faced by everyone, even though you are facing it at a younger age.

As a sibling, you will have many urges. You will be tempted to rush in, ahead of spouses. This is not good for anybody. You may feel that you know best, and you probably do, but it is important to respect your sibling's marriage and her children. She is trying to set an example for her children about many things—how to cope with illness, how married people take care of each other—so rushing in to take charge can give the children the wrong message.

Try not to take over, no matter how much you want to, unless your sibling is married to an idiot, in which case just get to work.

The best things my siblings did for me: gave me uncon-ditional love, prayed for me, made me laugh as only siblings and best friends can, told memories. Oh, and they baked.

Remember that there is something comforting in being with a sibling. Not with your spouse and your kids, just the siblings together. It is a warm feeling to be with the peo-ple you were a child with. Try to arrange sibling time for just yourselves. And if her childhood was filled with funny memories, go ahead and repeat them as often as the patient would like.

Helping the Family Member You Can't Stand

This is a challenging test. On holidays, you can hide in the crowd of family and avoid your least favorite relative. Not so when she has cancer. Can you put family before your own opinions and feelings? Can the patient do the same?

Let's say Aunt Betty has cancer and will be having extensive treatment. Aunt Betty is your husband's aunt, not yours. The rest of your husband's family lives elsewhere, your husband is on the road a lot; you are not. The problem is that Aunt Betty has been awful to you since your wed-ding day, when she started a fight with your mother about the seating plan.

If you can appear to be loving and caring, great. Maybe the illness has changed how you view Aunt Betty. Maybe it has changed how she behaves.

But if Aunt Betty drives you crazy and you behave badly when you're with her (or vice versa), find a way to help that does not involve a lot of contact. Nobody can fake it forever. If Aunt Betty is the kind of person who thinks she should always be driving the car, let's look at what can happen.

Her litany starts when she gets in your car. "You shouldn't let the rugs get so dirty. Don't go yet; can't you see my seatbelt isn't on? Forget it, go, I won't wear it anyway. I don't care if the car is beeping, I won't ruin this blouse with that seatbelt. Don't park in the garage, they charge a fortune. Park in the lot. It's a long walk but that will do you good. Just drop me off at the front door and park at the lot. No, I won't get you a validation sticker for the garage, because I want you to park in the lot. I know it's snowing, but I'm planning to pay for the parking, so I think it should be my decision, don't you? How hard could it be for you to clean the snow off your car? Oh, I forgot, you don't believe in cleaning your car."

How long can you do this? Not every day, or you will end up pulling over on the freeway and rolling Aunt Betty down a snow bank. That's not going to go down too well in your husband's family. Most likely.

Find something else to do for Aunt Betty, even if it's mowing her lawn. She probably won't appreciate it, but this isn't about her, or you, it's about your family and your positive role in it.

If you're stuck with a lot of contact, you're going to have to give Aunt Betty some boundaries. "It's hard for me to concentrate on my driving when we're talking, Aunt Betty. Let's wait until we get home." You might find this very difficult to do, but it is actually good for her. She needs boundaries and it will make her much easier to be around if she gets some. She may not love you for it, though. If you are helping her, if you can honestly say that you are doing what you believe you should be doing to help, nothing else matters.

When Your Friend's Child Has Cancer

Nothing is worse. You already know that. Be there, listen, help. Give them information about support groups, which they will love or loathe. Sit with them. Take care of the other kids. Listen, listen, listen. Then listen.

Chances are you'll outlive your parents and half of us will live longer than our spouses. Plenty of people can give you advice for situations like that, because so many people have been through it. But the illness of a child is beyond understanding. Stay close, very close, but remember that you really can't understand what they're going through.

I have heard people say to a parent of a sick child, "I know what you're going through. My grandmother had cancer." No, you don't know.

If you're uncomfortable about bringing the subject up, be open about that. I remember asking the mother of a child with cancer if she would mind if I brought it up, or if that would just make her think about it when she didn't want to. "I don't think about anything else," she said. "When you bring it up, it's already on my mind."

Parents go through very intense emotions during a child's illness, and they may unload them onto you. They may actually resent your healthy children. They may find being around healthy children impossible. They may be so angry at God or the world or medical science that they despair and are unable to feel much enthusiasm for life.

No situation will call on your friendship more than this one. Step in and help if you are a close friend. Don't wait for them to ask, just help.

Most of us know someone who has a sick child, but we're not close. Maybe your neighbor's child has cancer and you don't know each other well. You still want to help, and you have a few choices. You can try to contact the neighbor's close friends to see what you can do, or you can send a note to say that you are thinking of them.

There's really nothing in the world you can do that will make them feel better. If you keep trying, though, your love will help to sustain them until time can heal them.

When Your Friend's Parent Has Cancer

This is probably the most common relationship you'll find. More older people get cancer. Lots of elderly people die from it. If you're of a certain age, you may feel that parents start dropping like tomatoes.

No matter how old your friend is, no matter how old her parents are, she will suffer through their cancer. She will have to grow up in a way that she didn't have to before. Her parents may welcome her help, or they may not be able to cope with being dependent on a child. This may be everything they wanted to avoid.

Of course, they also might have trouble thinking she's competent. "I never trusted that kid to take out the garbage, and now she's driving my car?" is my favorite thing I've heard a parent say.

If your friend has an ill parent, let her be a child sometimes. Let her cry about it, complain about it, just like you did when you were teenagers.

If her parents die, set aside some time to get together and remember them. Tell stories about them. Let her laugh at the memories. If you are wondering how to help a good friend who has lost her parent, memories are by far the best gift to give.

When Your Child's Teacher Has Cancer

Some teachers will be very open about cancer so you can just follow all of the general advice in this book. Other teachers want to keep it a secret. They will buy a wig that is an exact duplicate of their own hair; they will put off the worst of the treatment until summertime. They don't want to discuss it and they don't want the kids finding out. I have even heard of parents who asked that the teacher not tell the children. I think the choice belongs to the teacher, not the parents, but your school may feel differently. Of course, the age of the children is a big factor. Kindergarteners don't need to know what a junior in high school deserves to know.

If the teacher prefers to be silent, whether you agree with this approach or not, you have to respect it. The problem is that the teacher really does need some help. I suggest going in and telling him that you would like to do some volunteer work for the classroom. Ask if there are any chores that need doing, during class time or not. If you can't do school-hour volunteering, ask if there are supplies that the class needs. Ask if you can help with anything at all. See? You never have to mention cancer. You're just being a helpful parent.

And remember that secrets are nearly impossible to keep, especially from children. They notice change, especially in the teachers and parents. I don't believe in a teacher going in and sobbing to the kids that she has cancer, but a simple explanation that she is sick and needs some medicine to get better is usually a good thing. Kids will always think something is really, really bad if adults have tried to keep it a secret.

When You're Estranged

If you have not spoken to someone because of a problem between you and you find out that they have cancer, proceed carefully. Like many important things in life, reconnecting can be delightful or it can be a powder keg. Much like a cousin's wedding.

Many people wish for reconciliation because they fear a person is dying. Before you take any steps, ask yourself if you're really ready for reconciliation. Ask if you can picture yourself taking at least half of the blame for whatever happened. Try to picture yourself rubbing his feet for him— could you do that if you harbor anger? Most of all, are you expecting forgiveness from an unforgiving person? Ask yourself if you're prepared for your efforts to be rejected.

Now you can either stay silent or try getting in touch. I think the best first step toward reconciliation is a phone call. A card or e-mail says, "I kind of want to reconcile, but I don't want to run the risk of talking to you." You be the judge—just be sure you are getting in touch for the right reason. If you feel guilty about how you behaved and don't want the guilt over this ex-friend haunting you, chances are you'll be more inclined to write a letter and avoid contact because the idea of the phone call makes you very anxious. That tells you that you are not really looking for reconciliation. If you write the letter, just make it an apology.

> **" I loved it when my friend . . . "**
>
> ". . . Took me to do something fun as soon as I was well enough. She let me decide what 'fun' means."
>
> ". . . Gave me a firm foam back wedge when I was recovering from surgery."
>
> ". . . Gave me a dense foam pad for the old mattress I had."

If you attempt to reconnect and feel that the patient wants nothing to do with you, you're going to have to stay away. He's facing a difficult challenge and does not need any more stresses in his life. In fact, keep quiet about the issue with everyone. Nobody needs to be focused on your anger at being rejected. Talk to another friend and let everyone focus on the patient, not you.

One big important note: If you're estranged because this person did something terrible to you, you have no duties whatsoever, and don't let anybody tell you that you do. An aunt or uncle who beat you gets no casseroles from you.

All the people who either don't know about this or never believed it happened will be giving you guilt trips. Please don't let them. I've seen it happen—adults who were badly abused as children being told to "make up with Dad before it's too late." But it was too late years ago, and you have no obligations. Seriously. Same goes for your husband's new wife (who was your maid of honor)—no obligations. Unless, of course, there are kids involved, in which case your obligation lies in the example you want to set for them.

When Your Coworker Has Cancer

A coworker with cancer presents a special challenge. There may be legal issues, privacy rules, sick leave, disability disputes, resentment about taking on the patient's workload. This section of the chapter covers the basic issues about helping someone living with cancer in the workplace. It does not help an employer to navigate the complex legal questions surrounding illness and employment.

The legal life of a cancer patient and her employer can be very messy. If you research this, be sure you're looking at current information. The Americans with Disabilities Act (ADA) is still relatively new, and I don't believe that anybody knows how it will work on your friend's individual case—whether she (or you) is the employee, the employer, the colleague, or the supervisor. The size of the company, the type of work, and the general benefits are all going to play a part.

If your friend has a small cancer for which she's going to have minor surgery and nothing else, good advice is "do yourself a favor and keep the details to yourself." That's right—don't tell anybody, not even her coworkers. This keeps life simple, especially if her job involves physical labor and she doesn't want her competence to be doubted.

If she's going to have chemotherapy, she may be productive or she may feel fatigued, or both. It's very rare nowadays that a cancer patient has to take a full-time leave of absence. That's reserved for very serious cases.

Tell her you're sorry to hear the news and want her to know that everyone is rooting for her. Spend time listening. If she has just been diagnosed, it's going to take time, maybe weeks, to find out what the treatment plan is going to be. Tell her to find out what she needs to know and then you can work together to address any issues.

Don't just suggest she go home! For everybody's sake, it's best to assume that life will be normal around the office. Deal with problems when you know they will happen, and don't get the whole place in a panic.

Most cancer patients who have chemotherapy will need more sick days than normal. If your workplace has a sick day pool, go ahead and contribute to it if you can, or encourage the company to start one. Find ways to keep her in the office loop. Keep her on the mailing list for things she would normally receive. Don't remove her in order not to worry her, because a dead stop to communication is going to worry her a whole lot more than a memo about trash in the lunchroom.

Have the person she gets along best with ask her how she would like people to communicate with her.

Sometimes an employee's illness can cause real concern and pain among colleagues and even clients and customers. It can help people to feel that they're helping. You might ask people to send her a song for her iPod. A book. A joke. A box of her favorite chocolates. Stationery with stamps on it. You might have each person who takes a shift of hers e-mail her to tell her what it was like. You can end every e-mail telling her that you miss her and hope she's back in full gear soon. Think about your colleague's family or children. Maybe they could use some new videos or games.

You may want to join in if someone is organizing meals or errands. You may want to be the one who does the organizing. Your colleague may be far away from family and have few friends outside of work.

Remember that you don't want to weaken your colleague. Don't say this: "Take as much time as you need, we'll do your work, don't give us a second thought." Cancer patients need goals, just as you do, and they need to feel needed, just as you do. "Let's work together to figure out what help you need and what you can do. Your responsibilities are important, and we want you to be as involved as you can be."

That may be surprising, but giving the patient a chore to do is a good and life-giving thing. Going too easy on the patient is destructive.

If you are the patient's employer and want to be generous, consider a temporary parking gift: a space close to the entry in the suburbs, a parking pass downtown. Make it simply clear that this is temporary, though. Consider what you might do for the employees who take on extra work for their sick coworker. I don't mean flowers; time off and money are always welcome.

✐

No matter how much you've learned so far, or how much experience you have with all of life's potholes, nobody can predict everything that will happen in each of your relationships. So next we'll cover a few unexpected developments that can happen.

CARE ALERT

The workplace may have legal potholes for the cancer patient and for the employer and the colleagues. Be kind, but think your actions through carefully, and if necessary, seek legal advice.

Chapter Ten

How Much Should I Help?

$\mathscr{L}$❤

YOU ARE EXHAUSTED. You have cooked, organized, driven, carpooled, and you're going to drop. Plus you feel guilty, because you think there's something wrong with you. You're out of energy and you're even running low on empathy and sympathy for your friend. Now maybe the holidays are coming up and you just know you're going to offer to help with the gift wrapping, or shipping or shopping.

Take comfort in the wisdom of my beloved friend Jane's rule: Nobody should receive more than a total of one month of meals. This one-month limit is true for widows and widowers, cancer patients, new parents. There are many other limits that can and should be placed on how far you're willing to go to help out. That's because people quickly become accustomed to your help and you have to be cautious about weakening them—yes, weakening them—by helping too much.

Every spouse knows that if you cook dinner once, your spouse will hate cooking more the next night. A spouse who takes out the garbage knows that next week the other one will be disappointed at having to do the job. Any muscle you don't use weakens, including the muscles that you use to cope with everyday life.

There will come a time when you have to begin backing off. How do you know when?

The answer should be that you'll just know, but that's hard. Maybe you're a generous person and it's easy for you to get in the habit of helping someone. Maybe you're not so generous. If you don't know, here's how you can calculate just how many things you should do for your friend.

The "How Much Should I Help" Calculator

When I first wrote this down I was kidding. Then I realized that it actually works pretty well. Give it a try and see what you think. You don't have to tell anybody that this is how you decided what you should do.

First, take one number from this list describing your friend:

1	Middle-aged person, with grown children, with healthy spouse
2	Middle-aged person, with grown children, no spouse available
3	Young person, married
4	Young person, single
5	Elderly person
5	Parents of a child with cancer, any age
5	Single parent with young children

Next, add one number from this list describing your relationship:

1	Acquaintance at work, church, school, neighborhood
2	Important acquaintance, such as children's teacher or close coworker
3	Friend you get together with once a month
4	In-laws or siblings
5	Best friend

Now multiply that number times the cancer stage, 1 through 4. The total is the number of things you should do—a meal, a lovely card, a visit, a ride—to be considered a great friend.

Say your best friend (5) is a single parent of children under twelve (5), which gives you a sum of 10. She has stage 3 breast cancer. Three times 10 is 30. You've got 30 things to do.

On the other hand, the usher at the synagogue is a married middle-aged man (1) plus he's an acquaintance (1) which gives you a sum of 2. He has Stage 1 prostate cancer. Two times one is two. You should do two things and be satisfied that you have done what you can or would be expected to.

Please don't tell anybody that I really think there is a way to calculate what you should do for a friend with cancer. This just accidentally happens to work.

Knowing When to Stop

Every cancer patient is different in how quickly they get back to normal. Everyone is different in how quickly they get hooked on help, too. At some point in your life you will visit a nonfavorite in-law weekly because she has cancer. Then you realize she thinks this is going to be a lifetime habit. You're going to have to tell her "I know you're feeling better but I would still love to see you often. Would once a month be too much?"

Or, you're going to know someone who becomes your best friend while she has cancer. You adore her and you love being best friends. Then it turns out that it was your big comfortable car she loved, and your generous gifts, and the hours of childcare you provided. You find this out when she plans a girl's weekend away and you're not invited. This person is going to hurt you, and you've experienced this before, haven't you? When you were the first kid in school to get a driver's license? High school never ends.

Most of the time, you're going to find that you've seen a friend through thick and thicker, and she's going to do the same for you someday. Most of the time, your friend can't wait to get back to normal, and is just incredibly grateful for everyone's help, support, and love.

But cancer does not make people angels, and if you find yourself starting to get worn out, take a break. Assess what you're doing. Decide if it's time to stop. Decide if you're draining the energy you need to take of your own family.

How Cancer Changes Life and Friendships

Treatment is over. Your friend is starting to feel pretty good again. She is trying to figure out how to face her fears of recurrence and she's doing pretty well at it. So what's next for your friendship?

Well, you can count on a few changes in your friend. In movies, cancer patients turn life upside down. In real life, cancer patients who throw their responsibilities to the wind like a seasick drunk are rare, fortunately, but it happens.

One place it can happen is in marriage. People will talk quietly about the number of couples who are divorced during treatment and usually blame a selfish man. Just as often, however, the wife decides to leave. She's thinking that if her time left is limited, she's not spending it with him. Again, it's uncommon, but not unknown. Divorce during cancer is shocking to everyone involved, but I haven't seen any actual numbers that show cancer patients getting divorced more often the general population.

More often the patient is worn out by the magical transformation everyone is waiting for. We are expected to be hang gliding, mountain climbing, running marathons. We are supposed to start our day with Pilates and end it running a fundraiser. What do we all really crave? A normal life.

Returning to "Normal" Life

People ask me this all the time: "Do you still do things you don't want to do?" Yes. I just don't do anything that I don't think is important. I don't go to meetings unless I have a contribution to make or I can learn something.

You may find your friend's editing of her life to be frustrating. Maybe there was something you always did together that she just doesn't want to do anymore. You may feel resentful; after all, you took care of her for months, doing everything she wanted to do; you may feel that she could do the same. Feel free to tell her that, but it may be tough to change her mind.

Another change I made is that now I don't have any friends I don't really like. You know the friends I mean. You worked together and ate lunch together sometimes. Then one of you left and now you want to get together again. You do that and discover that it was work that held you together. Still, you make a date for a Saturday lunch. One of you cancels. You reschedule and cancel again. You have become once-a-year friends, but you're still thinking like everyday friends.

> **" I loved it when my friend . . . "**
>
> ". . . Gave me a gift certificate for a local takeout service that delivers from many restaurants."
>
> ". . . Invited me to join in on gifts for other people, weddings and birthdays, so that I wouldn't have to shop."
>
> ". . . Set up a blog for me."
>
> ". . . Didn't mind that I never used the blog."

Cancer patients are given the gift of an edited life, so those friends will be in the past. It's kind of like the gift of losing your eyeglasses when your husband has started wearing sweatpants with a plaid shirt tucked in. It's all still there, you just don't deal with it. You fine-tune your time, your commitments, your friends.

If you have been a great friend through treatment, it doesn't mean you're going to be a great friend for life.

Sometimes, your friend gets stuck in Cancerland. He decides to devote his life to walking for a cure, running for a cure, talking about a cure. You're devoted to something else, like birth defects. He does not understand why you won't go on three-day walks or write checks when he walks. After all, he keeps giving you the cancer scarves and T-shirts that he earns.

All friends and friendships change and grow over time. Cancer accelerates that change. Sometimes you're the one who moves on, sometimes the friend is. You may or may not like the "new" friend who emerges at the other end of treatment. Maybe you like helping people more than you actually like your friend, and you'll move on to the next person who needs you. Maybe you've just changed, or he has.

Usually, though, your friend with cancer will be astonished at the love and support that will pour forth from a neighborhood, a family, a reading group, a faith. The friend who is fine for coffee but not for cancer will be left behind as the cancer patient learns to spend time and energy only on the most important things in life. As treatment ends, and recovery starts, this can foster and nourish the best and happiest parts of the mind.

The edited life is filled with the closest and most positive family and friends, mostly free of the rashes that people or things or experiences gave you before you knew how to edit.

Nobody is grateful to have cancer, but most people survive to lead a better, richer, and more fulfilling life. Patients can only hope to have learned enough from loved ones so that they know what to do when it's someone else's turn.

Epilogue

Today, Tomorrow, and Baseball

✒

I KEEP A picture of Lou Gehrig on my desk. When he was diagnosed with his devastating disease, he retired from baseball after a stunning career. He could no longer play. He gave his famous farewell speech on July 4, 1939, and I love to listen to the audio clips of it on *www.lougehrig .com*. You already know the highlight:

"Fans, for the past two weeks you have been reading about the bad break I got. Yet today I consider myself the luckiest man on the face of this earth."

He thanked the fans, and the Yankees, and the ground- skeepers, and even the rival Giants for being tough oppo- nents. He thanked his wonderful mother-in-law and father and mother and most of all, his wife. Then he said the most powerful expression of hope: "I may have had a tough break, but I have an awful lot to live for."

I can't imagine facing a disease that serious with that kind of courage. I was diagnosed with Stage III breast cancer in 2001, which is like having a cold sore compared to Lou Gehrig's disease. My children were thirteen and eight. Since then, I've had a few other cancer challenges, but I still believe that cancer has done nothing but lead to good things in my life. I feel very lucky.

I edited my life to the point that it is richer and fuller than ever before. I learned for the first time to look at the wonderful parts of my life and see "threads." I could see that for every problem in my life, there had been a thread that I could trace to something wonderful. Try it in your own life and I'll bet you find the same threads. It was terrible, for example, when my father slipped into a long illness—but it gave me treasured years of closeness with my sister Colette, as we drove to be with him every Sunday. And I didn't know I wanted to be a writer until I had cancer and sat down one night to jot down an e-mail about funny things I had seen that day in chemo.

Cancer trained me to learn the techniques of getting my mind around a problem. I learned to identify the period of shock and despair that can accompany a major challenge as a temporary thing. When bad things happen, I know in my heart that I will, with time, feel great again. In a moment of grief, that's awfully comforting.

Best of all, I was stunned by my friends and family. I had no idea that Laura and Jane were so filled with wisdom about my life with cancer, including that they hardly ever bring it up, or that my family could love me so openly and warmly, or that so many families would help us, or that so many people we hardly knew would become our friends.

Lou Gehrig didn't retire from living when he retired that day from the Yankees. He worked on programs to help troubled young people in New York. He inspires me, in how he lived, in how he faced his illness, and in how he died. Read his speech again—no self-pity, no complaint, just his profound gratitude for a full life. He described his terrible news and his heartbreaking retirement as "a bad break."

I look at his picture every day and every day I try to be like him. I'll never make it, of course. All of the little kids who admire baseball players with all of their hearts don't grow up to be pro ball players, and I don't pretend that I'll have Lou Gehrig's character or courage. But in the act of trying, a little bit every day, I feel renewed, refreshed, and reminded to try again tomorrow.

Sticking with baseball for a little bit, lifelong Red Sox fans like me know a thing or two about hope. Before 2004, when the Sox finally won the World Series for the first time since 1918, a lot of people made rash promises. "God, let them win and I can die tomorrow a happy girl. Let them win and I'll go to church every Sunday." We'd been sorely tested over the decades, and when they won again in 2007, we knew for sure that our hope was worth keeping for so long. I think we all felt that the world could end that day and everything would feel just fine.

Why do I feel the same hope about cancer? At a fast pace, cancer research is gaining on the disease. While it remains a challenge, new treatments and discoveries are giving new hope to many. When I was first diagnosed with a recurrence while writing this book, I assumed it would kill me. Now I assume it won't. For every treatment I try that works for a while, or doesn't, there will be a new one ahead soon. It doesn't mean that your friend is going to have the happy ending she deserves. But someday, sooner rather than later, cancer will be a manageable disease. I feel very excited for young doctors who are choosing to specialize in oncology. They're going to see incredible advances in their lifetimes and will be witness to one of the most exciting times in medical history.

It can be hard to hear about great advances when you're in the middle of your friend's treatment. The newspaper headlines will scream about a new discovery, then tell you it won't have any practical applications for a decade. Everybody who knows you have a friend with cancer will be e-mailing you the story, right? You'll have a full mailbox of forwarded stories, none of which mean anything for your friend. Sometimes, you'll even feel that your other friends don't want to hear anything about cancer and they want to dismiss your fears with a piece of good news from the headlines. Just keep telling yourself that they probably mean well.

I often think of the fears people had about strep throat before the introduction of penicillin. Strep could lead to scarlet fever or much worse, and many people died, until the miracle drug we now take for granted was discovered. Someday we'll view cancer in the same light: a disease that used to be life-threatening.

For now, for your friend, it remains a tremendous challenge, because the treatments are challenging and some kinds of cancer are devastating, silent killers. Future discoveries won't give her much comfort now. Sometimes the idea doesn't give me any comfort either; sometimes I want to go to bed and have the world wait on me while I languish away my life. But many things in life are like that. Many diseases make people feel that way. We cancer patients are lucky to have a disease that the world wants to cure.

Medicine has also made great leaps in limiting the side effects of treatment. Antinausea medicines have greatly diminished the burden of chemotherapy, as difficult as it still is. Yes, most of us still grow bald and don't feel so great, but it's not the nightmare it used to be.

Lou Gehrig's biggest legacy to me is that he teaches us the basic ingredient of happiness: gratitude. Gratitude for our lucky lives sustains us through the bumps in the road. It helps us to see the view, not just the bumps. Gratitude is a constant reminder of the gift of life and living. It's why so many people say that Thanksgiving Day is their favorite holiday; it makes us feel happy to be simply and deeply thankful.

I hope that you and your friend learn a lot together on your own journey through cancer. I hope it goes as smoothly as possible for you both, but also that you learn something from the inevitable bumps. I hope you both have much love, good health, and laughter along the way, which you will, because you are good friends.

Which makes you the luckiest people on the face of the earth.

Plans and Resources
for the Research Buddy

Research is going to help make choices, not find the one answer. If you start your quest for information believing that there is a definite answer to a complex question, you'll be looking forever. Cancer is not yet that kind of problem. The best research you can do is still going to be talking to the treatment team.

The LEVEL 1 Research Plan:
What to Do If All You Have Is a Pay Phone

1. Start by collecting the hospital or doctor's materials on your friend's kind of cancer. Take all of those pamphlets.

2. Call the Cancer Information Service (National Cancer Institute/National Institutes of Health, the primary government source for information) at 1-800-422-6237.

Ask them what they have, they'll send it, and it's all free. I got a package loaded with booklets, a video, and a catalog of other booklets. I called them on Thursday, it arrived on Monday.

3. Same thing with the American Cancer Society, at 1-800-227-2345. They can help you out with a lot more than information. They will try to find local sources for help with copayments, utility costs, medication costs; Road to Recovery volunteer drivers, who can take your friend to treatments; Peer Support volunteers, especially for breast and prostate cancer patients; and Look Good, Feel Better, which I have not gone to but is supposed to be a fun makeover with free samples. You can call ACS anytime. I tried them late at night and got a wonderful guy on the line—helpful, sensitive, supportive. Sorry, I didn't get his name or marital status.

You can stop right there if you have enough information now. Read something inspirational and you're done.

LEVEL 2 Research Plan:
When You Want to Go Beyond the Basics

Go online, which is the easiest way to learn a little more. If you're not online at home, head to the public library to use the Internet connection there. It's a good idea not to do Web searching at work. You have no privacy. You'll be amazed and maybe overwhelmed by the number of sites. There are thousands of sites around the world. I've pared the list to what I think are the most useful ones. By the time you're reading this, there are probably a bunch of new ones.

I recommend starting at a comprehensive place, like the American Cancer Society (*www.cancer.org*). Other good comprehensive sites: the government's National Institutes of Health site (*www.cancer.gov*), the National Comprehensive Cancer Network (*www.nccn.org*) and *www.oncology channel.com*. These sites all have sections on individual cancers. You can stop there, or you can follow their links to specific Web sites. (For breast cancer, for example, try *www .komen.org, www.imaginis.com, www.y-me.org, www.susan lovemd.com*, and *www.breastcancer.org*. Y-me.org also lists resources for free wigs.)

The more general medical sites also cover cancer, such as *www.webmd.com* and *www.medlineplus.com*.

If you want to go much deeper in research, try *www.asco .org*, which is the American Society of Clinical Oncology. The Association of Online Cancer Resources (*www.acor .org*) is a re-established center for Web sites. A mix of general information and medical updates can be found at *www .oncolink.com*.

If your friend is the research type, there is an interesting tool offered by the American Cancer Society online. You go to *www.cancer.org/profiletools* and click "Make Treatment Decisions." It will be best if you know the basic details of your pathology report. You click on your type of cancer, then you fill in the online questionnaire. They will ask you about your age, the size of your tumor, if you have lymph node involvement, all of the basics. The tool generates a report of treatment options with detailed information on each one, including side effects. The program is called the NexProfiler Treatment Option Tools for Cancer, and it's free. You do have to sign in.

Appendix B

Helpful Resources

Finding Clinical Trials

If you're looking for clinical trials, many of the sites in this section will give you information. But the first place to start is *www.cancer.gov* (or *www.clinicaltrials.gov*) and your own hospital.

A clinical trial usually means that a drug, or combination of drugs, is being tested on actual patients. If you're interested in clinical trials, either because your friend's cancer is advanced or he has an unhealthy generosity to help others, you will want to research each trial carefully before you urge him on. Don't do it without talking with the doctor. I also like to know who is sponsoring the trial. Since I don't know your hospital, I will just urge you to learn as much as possible about a trial before you do it. Be open to it, but cautious.

Online Community

You'll find plenty of information leading you to chat rooms, bulletin boards, and mailing lists (listservs) running at all hours. Since fear has a way of deepening at night, you might find it helpful to visit a chat room or online support group. But be very, very careful in all discussion groups, bulletin boards, and chat rooms. I don't just mean to protect your identity and never give your real name or location. I mean that there are plenty of people who visit these sites who have misinformation to spare. Most of the time they mean well, but sometimes they're peddling "cures." Just be careful. Don't take any action based on Internet information without talking to your doctor.

And, by the way, nobody yet has a "cure" for cancer. Be suspicious of any information that offers you a cure.

You may or may not have much in common with the people in any chat room or bulletin board. Sometimes I've visited a site and everybody is a young person facing aggressive cancer. I realize how lucky I am. Sometimes everybody has a benign lump but wants to talk about it. Sometimes they realize how lucky they are.

One of the biggest problems with online communities is that people get very huffy. Someone will say that they have Stage IV cancer with a small tumor and no lymph node involvement. Someone else gently says, "Guess what? You're probably not Stage IV!" thinking this will be received as the good news it is. But Madam Stage IV thinks you're saying she's ignorant and flames you, as they say. "I suppose you're a doctor?" she will sniff. If you're smart, you'll walk away without sending a reply. There are flame conversations that started on the Internet a decade ago, and you can still start them up by posting one controversial e-mail. This is fun but not helpful.

Very often, people go to a bulletin board or mailing list to ask for help in understanding what happened at their doctor's appointment. "My doctor said I have atypical cells. What does that mean?" Please call your doctor's office instead, or in addition to, whatever information you get. I understand the need at midnight to calm your fears, but I've seen an awful lot of bad information, such as "My mom had that and died in a week!"

If you live in a rural area with limited access to support groups, an online community may be just what your friend needs. That's especially true if he also has a rare form of cancer and feels that he can't relate well to all of the breast, skin, lung, and prostate folks out there. Of course, take precautions. Just. Be. Careful!

The best group for you will probably be for the kind of cancer your friend has. Ask the nurse to recommend one.

Then go to the National Cancer Institute Web site to look for national organizations that can help (*http://www.cancer .gov/cancertopics/factsheet/support/organizations*). You can search by type of cancer. You can also get a fact sheet by calling the Cancer Information Service at 1-800-4-CANCER or 1-800-422-6237. You can join an online support group at *www.thewellnesscommunity.org* and also on the American Cancer Society site at *www.acscsn.org/Forum/Discussion/ summary.html*

Cancer, Work, and Money

You can try *www.cancercare.org* for resources on financial help, because cancer can be a challenge if you're already having financial troubles. They list a lot of sources and give advice on finding local help. *Cancercare.org* also gives you resources for finding transportation. If you don't have Internet access, please remember that the hospital where you're being treated will have a resource person to help you. Please ask your doctor or nurse. The hospital itself may have someone to work with you on these issues.

Call the American Cancer Society, at 1-800-227-2345, day or night. They will try to find local resources to help with financial burdens.

Issues about work? Check out *www.cancerandcareers.org* for help ranging from employee rights to cosmetic help.

Your Friend Who Has a Teenager

Teenagers have special needs, and there's a great Web site to use as a resource: *www.canteen.org.au*. It's an Australian Web site and it's terrific. You name the category of teenager, they've got information.

Languages

Some of these Web sites and phone numbers will give you the option of speaking Spanish. (If you speak Spanish, Russian, Vietnamese, Tagalog, Korean, or Chinese, head to *www.y-me.org* for information on breast cancer. They've got printed materials and a Web site for you. They've got a hotline with interpreters for 150 languages. The English number is 800-221-2141.) Also take a look at *www.cancerindex.org*, which has a good list of resources available in several languages.

If you're helping someone who does not speak English, be sure to speak with the hospital's interpreter about research.

He or she may be more familiar with medical terms than even your best friend is and can be a great person to have on your team.

Web addresses change, as do services. Ask the hospital for more resources if you need them.

Lymphedema

If your friend develops lymphedema after cancer treatment, you'll be amazed by how little everyone knows about it. I think it needs a new name, like let's call it "cancer swelling," and that will get the world's attention. Of course, lymphedema has other causes, too. Since I'm not fond of research myself, I like easy, one-stop shopping. For lymphedema, go to *www.lymphnotes.com*. While a lot of the site is for people with primary lymphedema, not "cancer swelling," this site will link you to everything you need to know to help your friend.

Books

I wanted to spend as little time on cancer as possible, including learning about it. Also, I'm just stage III. If I am ever stage IV, which, God, if you're listening, I don't actually want to be, then this list might be different.

You will probably want a basic book about your friend's type of cancer. You can browse at the library or bookstore, but I would ask your nurse or doctor too. You can also check the Web sites for the national organization that is fighting this specific cancer. They often recommend books. There may be a learning center at your hospital that will have plenty of books to look at.

Books and articles are just a highly individual thing. Here are a few that I liked or loved that are about cancer in general.

- An article by Stephen Jay Gould called "The Median Isn't the Message," from *Bully for Brontosaurus* (W.W. Norton). If you do an online search for the title, you'll find the article. If you're worried about survival, read this.
- Lance Armstrong's *It's Not About the Bike* (Berkley). Inspiring, courageous, uplifting. Okay, so the marriage in the book doesn't have a happy ending, but I can put that aside and enjoy the rest of the story.
- *Cancer as a Turning Point: A Handbook for People with Cancer, Their Families and Health Professionals*, by Lawrence LeShan (Plume), which my oncologist brother-in-law, Rick Rosenberg, sent me.
- Margie Levine's *Surviving Cancer: One Woman's Story and Her Inspiring Program for Anyone Facing a Cancer*

Diagnosis (Broadway Books). Ms. Levine was facing a devastating diagnosis, which is probably not what you have, but this is very interesting anyway.

- Any book by Herbert Benson, M.D., a leading mind-body connection doctor (*www.mbmi.org*).

Think a bit before sending a cancer book. If there is one you know well, or have heard very good things about, go ahead and send it. Just follow two suggestions: Don't ask to have it back, and don't hound your friend to see if he has read it. When people give me a book, I tell them they will never see it again and if they want it back, please don't lend it to me. I am unreliable.

And every patient says that they had a stack of books and didn't always feel like reading about cancer. Some people read their books when treatment is all done.

To be truthful, I did not love cancer books, and I still don't. When someone gives me a cancer book, I don't think of it as a gift. I think it's homework. I appreciate the spirit of the gift, though.

Inspiration

Many people turn to inspirational reading. I received quite a few inspirational books, most of which I couldn't stand, but there were two that I treasured. My friend Roni Pick sent me *For Thou Art with Me*, by Rabbi Samuel Chiel and Henry Dreher (Daybreak/Rodale Books), a book that uses the Psalms to give you comfort and encouragement. My niece Christine sent me *Streams in the Desert*—by L. B. Cowman, updated by James Reimann (Zondervan)—which gives you a Bible passage and reflection for every day of a year. I looked up my birth date and it said, from Isaiah 52:12: "you will not leave in haste." Aaaah. This is a book that will carry you through as many days as you wish. If you're a person who likes short stories, you're going to love this approach.

I think you'll find inspiration everywhere around you, and most of it comes from sources that are not at all related to cancer or even illness. I am more moved and inspired by Holocaust survivor Viktor Frankl (read *Man's Search for Meaning*, Beacon Press, 2006) or by soaking in the spirits at Appomattox or Ellis Island, or reading the work of poet Langston Hughes.

My point? Seek your own inspiration. Viktor Frankl is mine for many reasons. For instance, while in Auschwitz, he wanted everyone in his group to think of something funny every day. I am very inspired by that. If he could laugh in Auschwitz, well then surely I can laugh in the United States.

However many books you get, please, please, please remember: If you're feeling awful, you're supposed to call the doctor. This isn't a cold, so don't try to diagnose yourself, even using a good book.

Support

Of course your family and friends are your best support. But many people find that it's comforting to go someplace and talk about cancer or treatment, where everybody there is in the same boat. Your hospital may have good support groups or therapy available if these would be helpful for you. You may want to start there rather than invest a lot of time and energy in a search for a good match with a therapist, unless you can get some very good referrals.

You're not seeking this support because you're nuts. You're seeking it because it can help you to be stronger, which is going to help you cope, which is going to improve your body.

Many people swear by the Wellness Community Centers for all kinds of support. Call 1-888-793-WELL or *www.wellness-community.org* to see if there is one near you. They offer many free services and support groups.

For information on free mammograms, cervical cancer tests (Pap smears), and other screening programs, call the Centers for Disease Control at 1-888-842-6355. They'll give you a telephone number for your state.

If you don't have computer access at home, and you can go to a public library, you may be able to get help using the Internet there. Your hospital may also have online research facilities for you to use. If none of this works, be sure to tell your doctor or nurse that you have unanswered questions.

Index

About the Author

MONIQUE DOYLE SPENCER is a breast cancer survivor and a friend and daughter to many people who have confronted the disease in its many forms. She wrote about her experience with humor and wit in *The Courage Muscle: A Chicken's Guide to Living with Breast Cancer*, which gained attention from hospitals, doctors, patients, and *BusinessWeek*. She's a regular on the speaking circuit and is frequently featured in the *Boston Globe*'s op-ed pages. As a speaker, she is often asked what a person can do as the friend of someone with cancer. A PR consultant, she lives in Brookline, Massachusetts, with her husband and two daughters.